CONTENTS

INTRODUCTION

PEOPLE CAN BE CLASSIFIED INTO TWO CATEGORIES— THOSE WHO HAVE BACK PAIN AND THOSE WHO WILL GET BACK PAIN.

During my years as a naprapath treating neuromusculo-skeletal conditions, the same question from patients pops up time after time: "Is it really necessary to stretch? Do I have to?"

The answer is neither yes nor no. Have to? Well, do you have to brush your teeth? No, not really, but most of us are fairly aware of the consequences if we don't. Sadly enough, we do not see the consequences of neglecting to stretch and take care of our bodies until we are reminded by pain in all kinds of places.

We may not even realize then that the pain is connected to our behavior. Until now, our bodies have not required maintenance, so why is the pain starting now? Would we have been as surprised by a cavity if we hadn't brushed our teeth for the past six months? You save up for pain. The body does not forget what you have been up to the last 20 years.

So, do we need to stretch? I believe that stretching and exercise are part of the body's daily maintenance. It should be no different than the habit of brushing our teeth.

Stretching in one form or another has been habitually practiced by man and animal alike. Consider a cat or a dog that is waking up. They stretch their shoulder and hip muscles before starting any activity. Is it possible that we have lost this animal instinct as our lives have demanded less and less activity from us? Although this might be true, the instinct is still there. When we yawn in the morning, we tend to stretch our arms up and out and to bend our backs.

The last 10 years of my time as a gymnast were a real pain. My back constantly ached. I even got to experience throwing my back out before that career was over. As a gymnast, and a flexible one at that, I really thought I was an authority on muscles and flexibility. Later, during my studies to become a naprapath, I found out about muscles I never even knew existed.

However, even during my student years, my back continued to hurt. Regardless of the treatment, the pain only improved marginally. After a while, I started to feel some improvement from consistently stretching a particular muscle. I made up my mind that the muscle on the other side of my body should be just as soft and flexible. I started to see results. Nowadays, my back never bothers me. If I start to feel pain after training or negligence, I just stretch the same muscle that I stretched before. When I am done, the pain is gone. In retrospect, I sometimes wonder how I would have performed as a gymnast if I knew then what I know now. The health of a single muscle made a world of difference.

This is the experience that I try to pass on to my patients. Every patient gets one exercise to do at home. I can easily tell who has done the homework and who has forgotten to do it. By working together, we quickly reach the desired results of less pain and increased mobility.

Stretching books and magazines are often filled with miracle stretches. Sadly enough, they do not address the real reason why we need to stretch. The exercises in the articles are often wrong or dangerous, and the instructions for performing them are often incomplete, hard to follow, or nonexistent.

This book is a tool, and like all other tools, it should be handled carefully. Read it through and study the pictures thoroughly. The exercises work, but only if you do them correctly.

PRESCRIPTIVE STRETCHING

KRISTIAN BERG

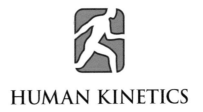

HUMAN KINETICS

Library of Congress Cataloging-in-Publication Data

Berg, Kristian, 1964-
  Prescriptive stretching / Kristian Berg.
      p. cm.
  Includes bibliographical references and index.
  ISBN-13: 978-0-7360-9936-3 (soft cover)
  ISBN-10: 0-7360-9936-0 (soft cover)
  1. Stretching exercises. 2. Exercise--Physiological aspects. 3.
Physical fitness. I. Title.

  RA781.63.B47 2011
  613.7'182--dc22

                                                    2010046614
  ISBN-10: 0-7360-9936-0 (print)
  ISBN-13: 978-0-7360-9936-3 (print)

Copyright © 2011 by Kristian Berg

This book is a revised edition of *Stora Stretchboken,* published in 1994 by Fitnessförlaget.

Acquisitions Editor: Tom Heine; **Managing Editor:** Julie Marx Goodreau; **Assistant Editor:** Elizabeth Evans; **Copyeditor:** Joy Wotherspoon; **Graphic Designer:** Jessica Stigsdotter Axberg; **Graphic Artist:** Kim McFarland; **Cover Designer:** Keith Blomberg; **Illustrator:** Erik Beijer; **Printer:** United Graphics

Human Kinetics books are available at special discounts for bulk purchase. Special editions or book excerpts can also be created to specification. For details, contact the Special Sales Manager at Human Kinetics.

Printed in the United States of America   10   9   8   7   6   5   4   3   2   1

The paper in this book is certified under a sustainable forestry program.

Human Kinetics
Web site: www.HumanKinetics.com

United States: Human Kinetics
P.O. Box 5076
Champaign, IL 61825-5076
800-747-4457
e-mail: humank@hkusa.com

Canada: Human Kinetics
475 Devonshire Road Unit 100
Windsor, ON N8Y 2L5
800-465-7301 (in Canada only)
e-mail: info@hkcanada.com

Europe: Human Kinetics
107 Bradford Road
Stanningley
Leeds LS28 6AT, United Kingdom
+44 (0) 113 255 5665
e-mail: hk@hkeurope.com

Australia: Human Kinetics
57A Price Avenue
Lower Mitcham, South Australia 5062
08 8372 0999
e-mail: info@hkaustralia.com

New Zealand: Human Kinetics
P.O. Box 80
Torrens Park, South Australia 5062
0800 222 062
e-mail: info@hknewzealand.com

E5249

MUSCLES AND BONES OF THE HUMAN BODY

The Latin names for muscles usually describe what they look like or what their functions are. For this reason, it is useful to learn the Latin terms. Let's take the example of the levator scapulae muscle. *Levator* stems from *levatio,* which means *raise.* You can see this origin of the modern word *elevator. Scapula* is the Latin word for the shoulder blade. The examples are endless. You can easily deduce the use and position of the muscles if you are familiar with some Latin terminology. Here are some examples:

Abdominis = Abdomen

Abductor = Outward moving

Adductor = Inward moving

Antebrachii = Forearm

Anterior = Front side

Bi = Two

Brachii = Upper arm

Brevis = Short

Caput = Head

Dorsum = Back

Externus = Outer/External

Extensor = Muscle that extends/ straightens

Femoris = Thigh

Flexor = Muscle that bends

Infra = Below

Internus = Inner/internal

Lateralis = Toward the side

Levator = Muscle that raises

Longus = Long

Magnus/Major = Large/greater than

Minimus/Minor = Small/lesser than

Musculus = Muscle

Musculi = Muscles

Obliquus = Slanted

Posterior = Back side

Processus = Process

Rectus = Straight

Spinae = Spine

Supra = Above

Tri = Three

A NOTE ABOUT THE STRETCHES
Throughout the book we show all of the stretches on the right side.
Naturally, you need to stretch the left side as well.

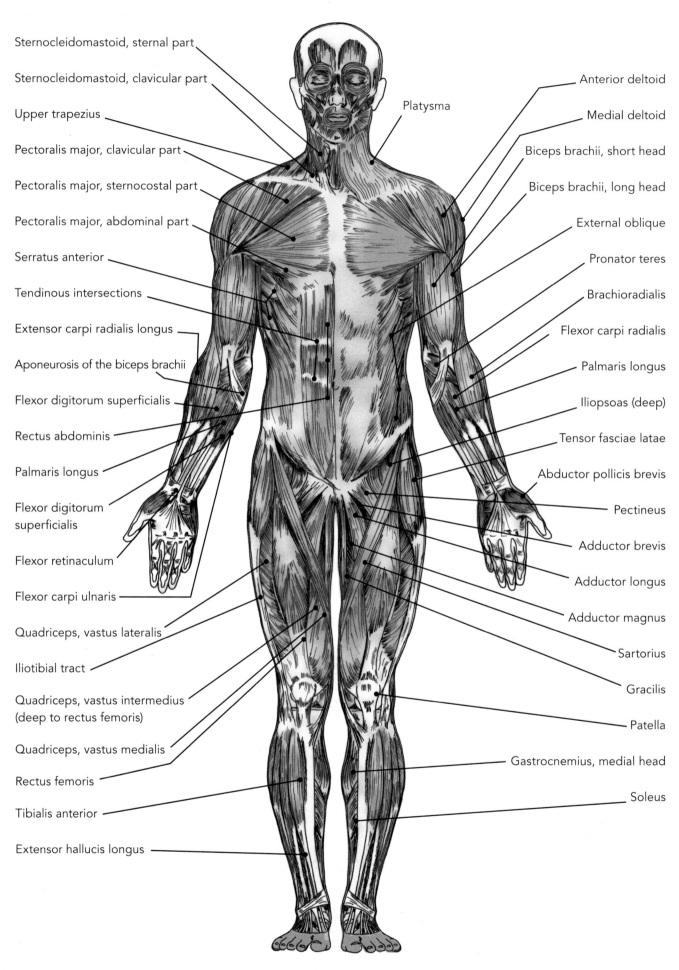

Sternocleidomastoid, sternal part

Sternocleidomastoid, clavicular part

Upper trapezius

Pectoralis major, clavicular part

Pectoralis major, sternocostal part

Pectoralis major, abdominal part

Serratus anterior

Tendinous intersections

Extensor carpi radialis longus

Aponeurosis of the biceps brachii

Flexor digitorum superficialis

Rectus abdominis

Palmaris longus

Flexor digitorum superficialis

Flexor retinaculum

Flexor carpi ulnaris

Quadriceps, vastus lateralis

Iliotibial tract

Quadriceps, vastus intermedius (deep to rectus femoris)

Quadriceps, vastus medialis

Rectus femoris

Tibialis anterior

Extensor hallucis longus

Platysma

Anterior deltoid

Medial deltoid

Biceps brachii, short head

Biceps brachii, long head

External oblique

Pronator teres

Brachioradialis

Flexor carpi radialis

Palmaris longus

Iliopsoas (deep)

Tensor fasciae latae

Abductor pollicis brevis

Pectineus

Adductor brevis

Adductor longus

Adductor magnus

Sartorius

Gracilis

Patella

Gastrocnemius, medial head

Soleus

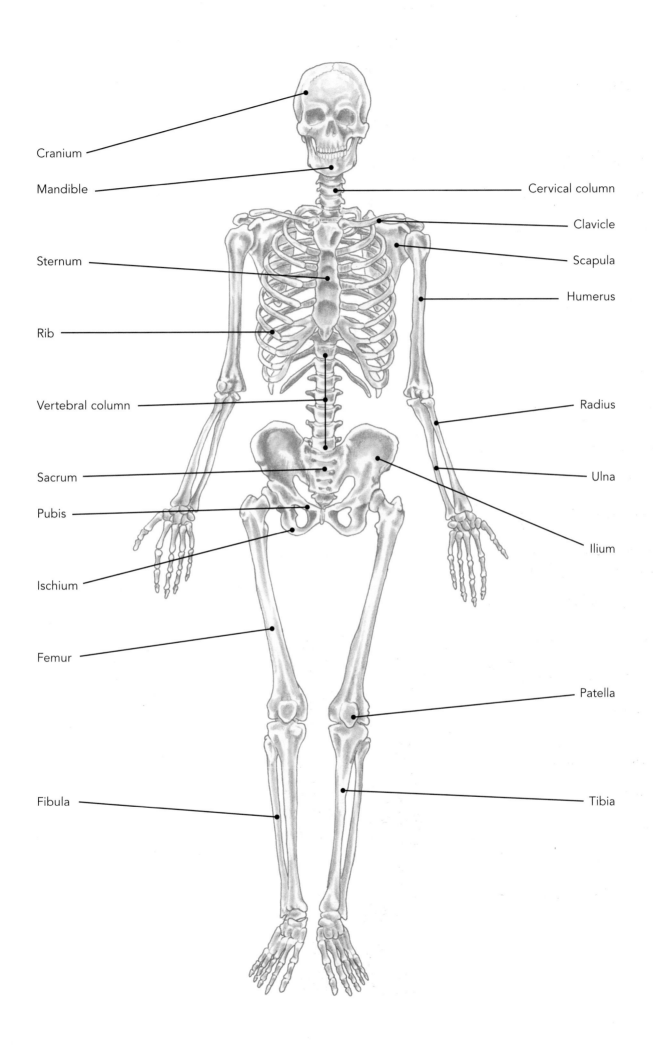

Cranium

Mandible

Cervical column

Clavicle

Scapula

Sternum

Humerus

Rib

Vertebral column

Radius

Sacrum

Ulna

Pubis

Ischium

Ilium

Femur

Patella

Fibula

Tibia

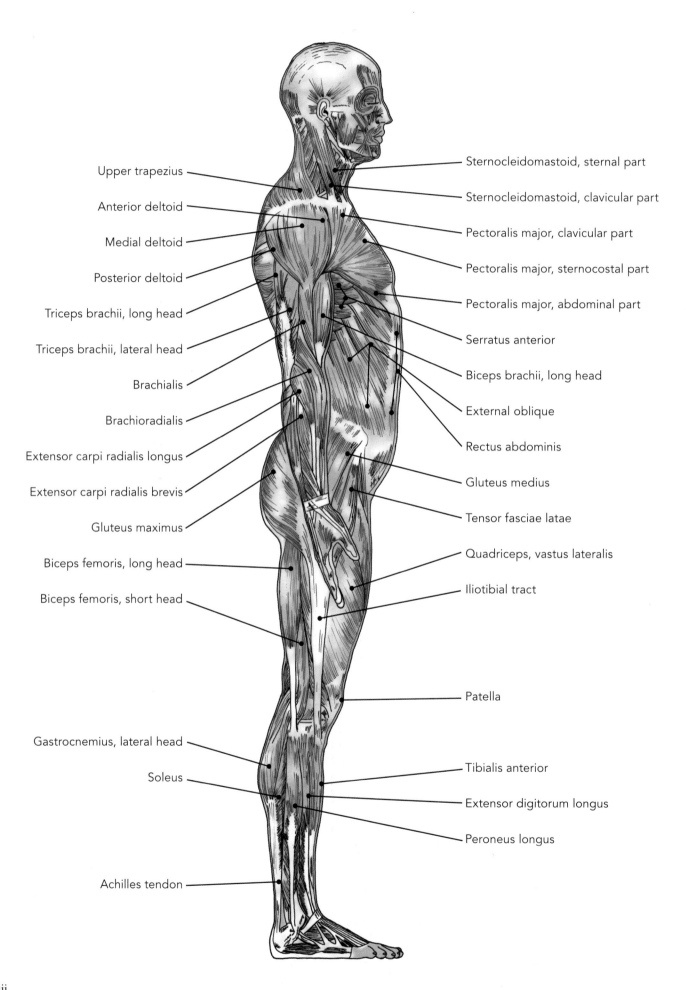

Upper trapezius

Anterior deltoid

Medial deltoid

Posterior deltoid

Triceps brachii, long head

Triceps brachii, lateral head

Brachialis

Brachioradialis

Extensor carpi radialis longus

Extensor carpi radialis brevis

Gluteus maximus

Biceps femoris, long head

Biceps femoris, short head

Gastrocnemius, lateral head

Soleus

Achilles tendon

Sternocleidomastoid, sternal part

Sternocleidomastoid, clavicular part

Pectoralis major, clavicular part

Pectoralis major, sternocostal part

Pectoralis major, abdominal part

Serratus anterior

Biceps brachii, long head

External oblique

Rectus abdominis

Gluteus medius

Tensor fasciae latae

Quadriceps, vastus lateralis

Iliotibial tract

Patella

Tibialis anterior

Extensor digitorum longus

Peroneus longus

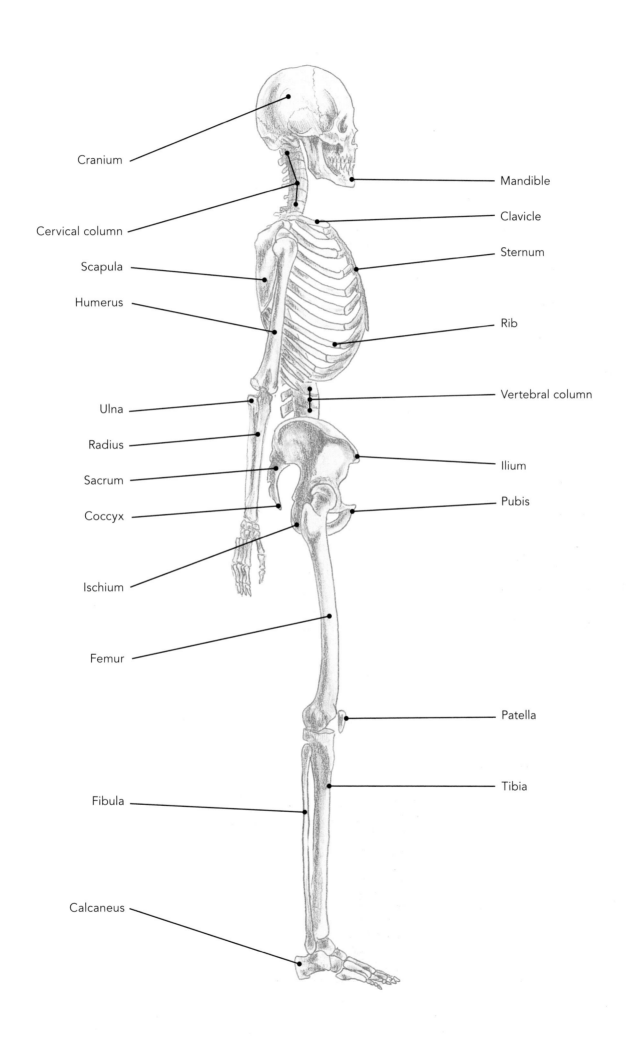

Cranium

Cervical column

Scapula

Humerus

Ulna

Radius

Sacrum

Coccyx

Ischium

Femur

Fibula

Calcaneus

Mandible

Clavicle

Sternum

Rib

Vertebral column

Ilium

Pubis

Patella

Tibia

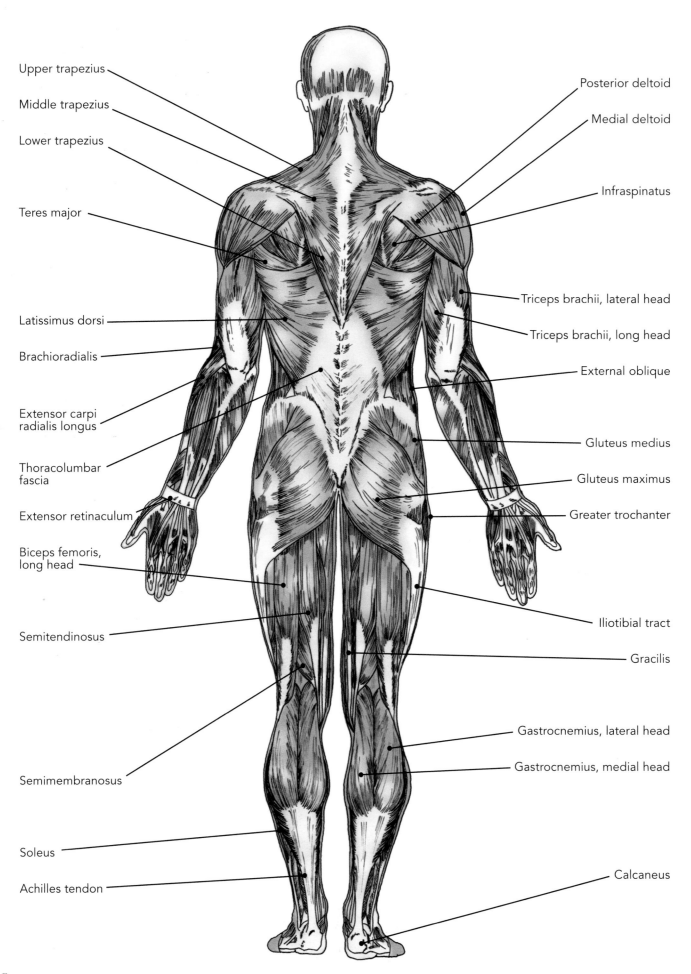

Upper trapezius

Middle trapezius

Lower trapezius

Teres major

Latissimus dorsi

Brachioradialis

Extensor carpi
radialis longus

Thoracolumbar
fascia

Extensor retinaculum

Biceps femoris,
long head

Semitendinosus

Semimembranosus

Soleus

Achilles tendon

Posterior deltoid

Medial deltoid

Infraspinatus

Triceps brachii, lateral head

Triceps brachii, long head

External oblique

Gluteus medius

Gluteus maximus

Greater trochanter

Iliotibial tract

Gracilis

Gastrocnemius, lateral head

Gastrocnemius, medial head

Calcaneus

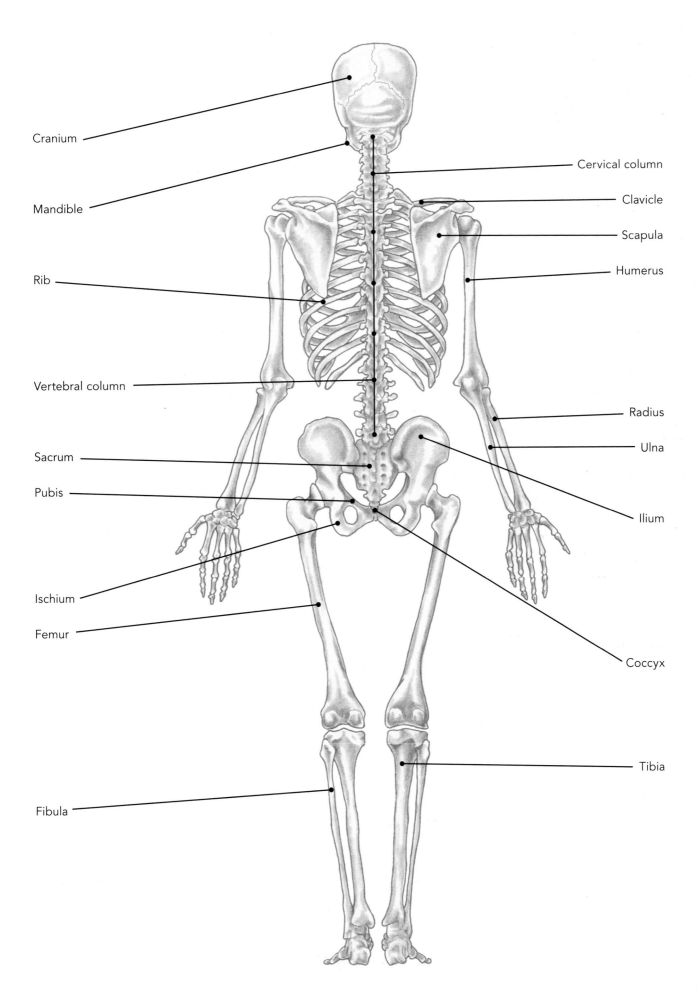

Cranium

Mandible

Rib

Vertebral column

Sacrum

Pubis

Ischium

Femur

Fibula

Cervical column

Clavicle

Scapula

Humerus

Radius

Ulna

Ilium

Coccyx

Tibia

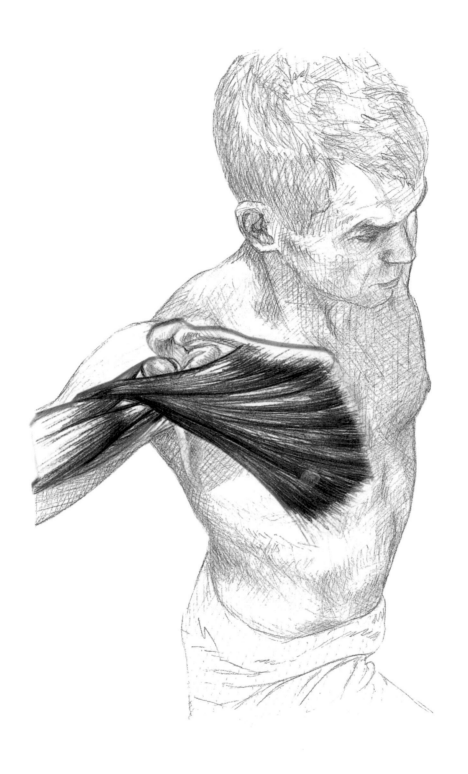

STRETCHING
FUNDAMENTALS

PHYSIOLOGY

The human body is an amazing creation. A variety of systems ensure that everything works just as it was intended to, from vision, hearing, and circulation to the kidneys and the heart. One of the most important systems is the motor system, which controls movement, flexibility, strength, coordination, and balance.

This group of systems contains the bones, joints, and the skeletal muscles, which all need resistance to stay healthy throughout your entire life. We put all the building blocks in place as children and must maintain them as adults.

When we move, the blood flow increases to the affected area. The blood carries oxygen and other nutrients that the muscles need. It also increases the temperature, making the muscles pliant. Muscle resistance stimulates growth so that the body will be stronger for the next exercise bout. You should increase resistance incrementally so that your body has a chance to adjust. If you increase the resistance too quickly, you will overload your muscles. All forms of overloading are relative. They can include walking for too long, walking too often, or lifting something too heavy. You can even overload your muscles by sitting too much.

Increasing resistance incrementally is important for preventing injury during any kind of training or stretching. Even if you don't feel like taking it easy, your body registers everything you do. If you do too much of something over a short period of time, your body will let you know by registering pain.

THE MUSCULAR SYSTEM

The body contains about 300 skeletal muscles that are designed to create movement in the joints. Think of these muscles as stretched rubber bands. When a muscle goes into action, it pulls in like a rubber band. The more elastic your muscles are, the smoother your movements will be.

Muscles that never are asked to do any work do not get stronger during rest. Instead, they become tight and shortened, which cause pain. When you need the muscles, they will become tired easily because they are not used to performing any work. As a result, you may throw your back out while performing a simple, everyday task, such as moving a chair.

The body needs balance. When they are used, the muscles in the front of the body pull everything forward. If these muscles are shortened, a hunched-over posture will result. Therefore, in order to stand up straight, the muscles in the back need to be either equally long and strong or short and weak. In the best scenario, the muscles on the front and back of the

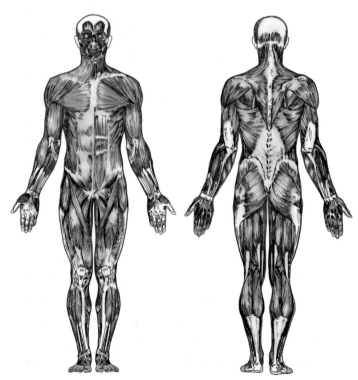

The human body contains 300 skeletal muscles.

body are equally elastic, requiring less energy to stay balanced.

The relationship between the muscles on the different sides of the body (front and back or right and left) is very important for both performance and well-being.

Muscles that are repeatedly tightened (for example, during stress) will lose their elasticity and stiffen over time, since blood circulation decreases as we move less.

ANTAGONISTS

An antagonist is a muscle that creates the movement opposite to that of the muscle currently working or stretching. If the muscle that you are stretching bends the elbow, then its antagonist straightens the elbow. Therefore, when you execute a movement using a set of muscles, tight antagonists will provide resistance to that movement. If you are aware of the antagonists that cause most of the trouble, you can become much more efficient. For example, during running, you bring the leg forward using the hip flexors and the quads. The muscles on the back side of the thigh that move the leg backward will get stretched out as the leg moves forward. If these muscles are tight, they will hinder the movement. Stretching these muscles before running makes the activity more efficient.

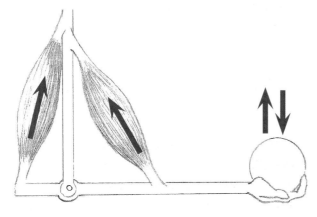

Red will raise the ball and blue will lower the ball. They work in opposite directions, so they are antagonists.

SHORTENED MUSCLES AND TRIGGER POINTS

When the muscles work, they produce by-products. One of these by-products is called lactic acid. Anyone who has carried something for a long time has felt the effects of lactic acid. At first, you feel a burn in the muscle. As you get more and more tired, the area actually starts to hurt. When you let go of what you were carrying, the pain dissipates because blood removes the lactic acid from the muscle.

If you continually tighten your muscles, you create the problem of too much lactic acid. Nowadays, due to stress, we continually tighten the muscles in the neck and shoulder region. This practice also contributes to poor posture, which can be caused by weak muscles or by an adaptation of the body to shortened muscles. This bad habit also creates increased resistance when standing or sitting with correct posture. This resistance can shorten the muscles even further.

Trigger points can best be described as knots in the muscle that can vary in size from that of a rice kernel to that of a pea. Trigger points can cause pain, both locally and in other areas of the body. They can be either active or latent. For example, an active trigger point in the shoulder area, the trapezius muscle, can cause headaches either around the ears or near the forehead and eyes. A latent trigger point in the same area causes similar pain when pressed.

Trigger points appear in muscles that are shortened and tightened in a static manner, thereby producing lactic acid. They can also appear in muscles that work too much without any rest. Trigger points can create pain that radiates down the arms and into the hands or legs. They can also cause local pain in the back. Some trigger points will always cause pain in the same location for all people. These help us find the cause of the pain. Stretching is a good way to remove trigger points or to make active ones latent.

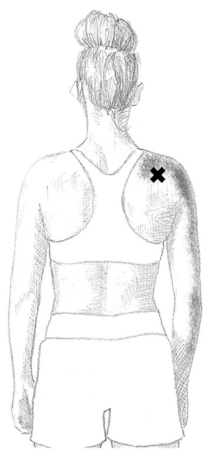

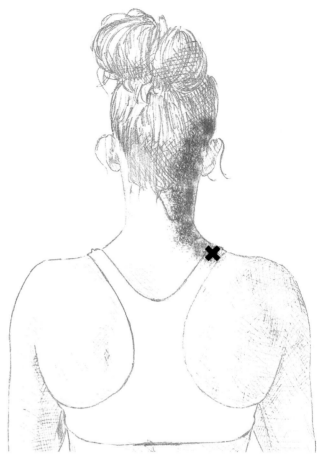

The X marks the placement of the trigger point, while the color indicates the area where pain might be felt. The entire area may not necessarily be affected.

The most common headache stems from a trigger point in the upper part of the trapezius muscle.

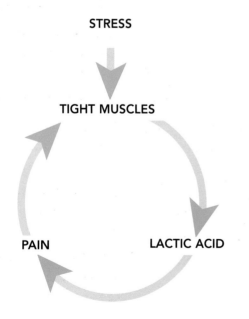

STRESS

TIGHT MUSCLES

PAIN

LACTIC ACID

Following are the most common reasons for shortened muscles and trigger points:

- Stress
- Bad posture
- Static load
- Sitting (general inactivity)
- Sleeping for an extended time in an uncomfortable position
- Repeated movements (especially above the head)
- Training with poor technique
- Sitting with crossed legs
- Habitually carrying a bag on the same shoulder
- Feeling cold

THE SKELETAL SYSTEM

Everything in the body hangs on the skeleton, from the muscles and the lungs to the liver and intestines. If the skeleton proves to be too brittle, everything falls apart. Movement and loading stimulates the skeleton to strengthen and rebuild itself during the night to prepare for the needs of the following day. However, a sedentary life does not give the skeleton a reason to get stronger. Inactivity causes the skeleton to stop rebuilding, becoming thinner and less durable. Regrettably, your time to build a strong skeleton is limited. This process occurs until age 25, but after that, it is very difficult to substantially strengthen the skeleton. So, make sure your kids get out and move around instead of sitting in front of the computer or the television all day. The skeleton and the body are created for work, not for rest.

When you fracture a bone, the body heals it and then adds a layer of tissue on top to decrease the chance of another break.

JOINTS

Your joints, or the connection between two bones, might be the most sensitive part of the motor system. The ends of your bones are covered with cartilage that dampens vibrations and lessens friction. Like the rest of the skeleton, the cartilage needs to be loaded. It thickens during the first years of our lives. The more often cartilage is loaded, the thicker and more functional it becomes.

A door that is constantly opened and closed but is never greased will start to squeak. The same is true for our joints, which need maintenance and movement. Loading is the best way to care for your joints. Moving a joint though its entire range of motion stimulates it and makes it more cooperative the next time it is used.

Joints that are not used stiffen up. After only 12 hours in a cast, the mobility of the elbow joint decreases to 30 percent of its original function.

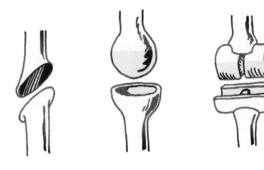

The plane joint, the ball-and-socket joint, and the hinge joint are three of the six kinds of joints in the body. The shape of the joint determines the movements that it can perform.

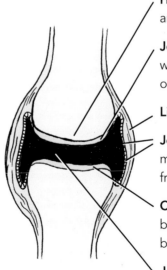

Head of a joint. Usually round and covered with cartilage

Joint cavity. Flatter, covered with cartilage; fits the head of the bone

Ligament. Stabilizes the joint

Joint capsule. Restricts movement and provides protection from dirt and bacteria

Cartilage. Lessens friction between the head of the bone and the cavity

Joint fluid. Lessens friction and wear and tear to the joint; transports nutrients

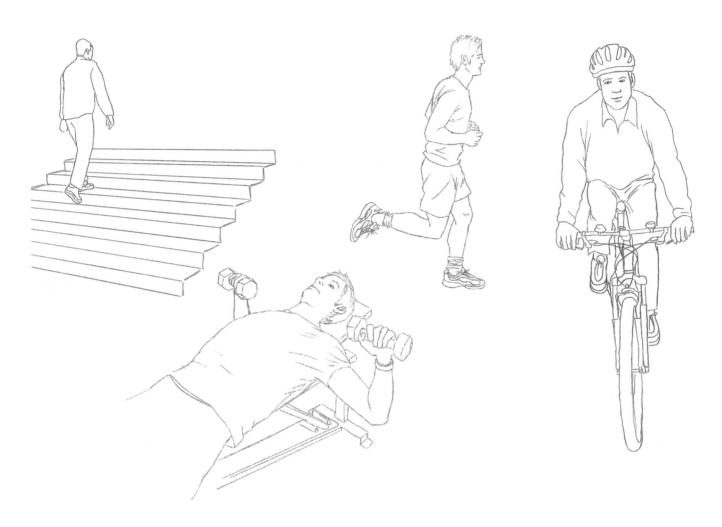

Moving for approximately 30 minutes per day is the best way to protect your back and your body as a whole.

GET MOVING!

Regrettably, modern life provides conveniences, such as chairs, escalators, and elevators, which rob the body of the stimulus that it needs. Resting all day does not save the body from suffering and trouble. Instead, it decreases the body's chances to feel good. Our bodies are built to walk for weeks on end, preferably with a backpack. This has always been the case for both young and old people.

A good way to keep track of how much you move is to get a pedometer that counts every step you take. However, the rest of your body needs to work just as much as the legs do. All your joints and muscles need daily activity to feel good. When the body feels good, you feel good.

Pedometer	
Fewer than 1,000 steps:	You have got to get off the couch.
1,000 to 3,000 steps:	Your lack of movement is dangerous to your health.
3,000 to 5,000 steps:	Better, but now try to go outside.
5,000 to 10,000 steps:	Good, you are almost there. Just a couple more steps.
More than 10,000 steps:	Good work! Now the real health benefits will start to show up.

RESULTS OF INACTIVITY

Heart

If the heart is never challenged, it will do as little work as possible, preventing it from going the extra distance when you need it to. A weak heart also hampers your circulation.

Muscles

Muscles that are not used waste away, preventing them from performing well when you need them. The tendons become fragile and can easily tear with sudden movements. Muscles that are not maintained lose their elasticity and become stiff.

Joints

During youth, the body's cartilage is enhanced by movement. If you were inactive as a kid, your cartilage will be thinner than it would be had you been active. Thin cartilage increases the risk of arthritis.

Bones

Just like cartilage, bones get stronger when they are loaded. The main reason for a brittle skeleton is inactivity. Osteoporosis is the most common reason for fractures among elderly people.

Circulation

Inactivity causes the capillaries, or small blood vessels, to withdraw, preventing distribution of oxygen to your muscles and other tissues.

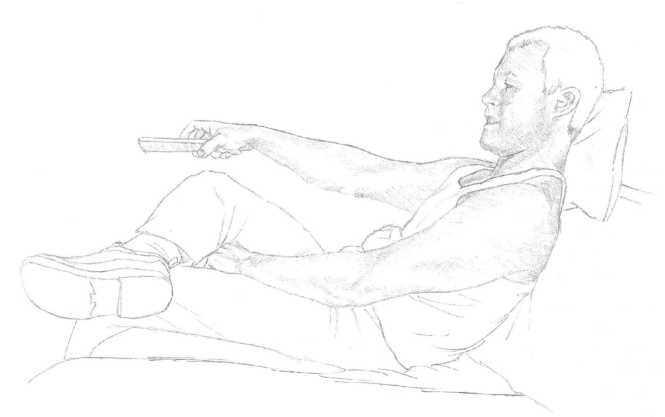

Being a little bit lazy is not really dangerous as long as you incorporate some activity into your daily life.

WHY STRETCH?

A lot of research has been done on stretching. Sadly, much of it has not been done well. However, lately some well-designed research has shown that consistent stretching increases strength and decreases pain. Some studies even indicate that you can use stretching to prevent injuries in different sports.

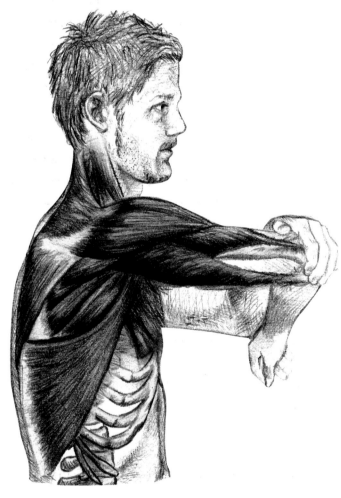

A stretch of the infraspinatus muscle, which can reduce pain in the front of the shoulder.

Some findings indicate that the chemical components of muscles are altered by pain. Researchers feel that stretching increases blood flow to the muscle, causing it to relax more. As the circulation increases, the blood washes substances that cause pain out of the muscle, thereby decreasing the pain.

Certain studies show that stretching increases mobility, but this depends on the technique used and the person's age. Other studies indicate that stretching helps people tolerate pain better.

Even studies that are less scientific show how stretching increases mobility. For example, in cases of acute immobility in the neck, stretching can immediately improve the range of motion and decrease the level of pain. However, it is very difficult to scientifically determine whether stretching makes the muscle longer or more relaxed. Some research shows that stretching makes muscles stronger, especially the antagonist of the muscle being stretched. This is of particular interest for strength training. If you train your latissimus dorsi, stretching the chest muscle creates gains in both mobility and strength.

HOW TO STRETCH

Using the wrong technique during stretching can waste your time and increase your risk of injury. Be aware of the fact that when you stretch a muscle, you will also perform at least one action that is directly opposite to what the muscle does as it works (contracts).

If the function of the muscle is to bend the elbow, you need to straighten the elbow in order to stretch it. If a muscle flexes the hip, straightens the knee, or increases the arch in your lower back, in order to achieve a stretch, you need to extend the hip, bend the knee, or lessen the arch of the back. Performing only one of these actions will not yield the desired stretch. It can also increase the mobility in the joints too much, which can lead to injury. Follow the instructions for stretches closely in order to exercise effectively and safely.

FOUR MAIN PRINCIPLES

To stretch safely, you must adhere to the four main principles of avoiding pain, stretching slowly, stretching the right muscle, and working only the necessary joints and muscles. These guidelines are designed to make your stretching safer and more effective and to increase your awareness of your body.

Avoid Pain

If you stretch carefully, your muscles will react in the desired manner. If you force the stretch, your muscles will not want to cooperate. If you stretch to the point of pain, your body's defense mechanisms will kick in, thinking something dangerous might be going on. When muscles register pain, they try to protect themselves by contracting. This is the opposite of you want to achieve by stretching. Of course, very slight pain during a stretch can feel good if the discomfort does not spread to the body. However, you must be able to distinguish between the burn of stretching and pain that will lead to an injury.

Stretch Slowly

If you throw your arms or legs out during the stretch, the muscle will stretch too fast. This makes the body think that the muscle is about to get torn or injured. Once again, it will try to protect the muscle by contracting it, preventing you from reaching your goal.

Stretch the Correct Muscle

Although this might sound obvious, you must use correct technique in order to follow this rule. Movement that goes a couple of degrees in the wrong direction can mean the difference between stretching the muscle and pulling on the joint capsule or similarly harming the body. To save your body and valuable time, it is important to do things right!

Avoid Affecting Other Muscles and Joints

Stretching that is careless or poorly done can negatively affect other muscles and joints, actually worsening your condition. This common mistake is the main reason why some people consider stretching worthless or painful.

Four Main Principles

Avoid pain.

Stretch slowly.

Stretch the correct muscle.

Avoid affecting other muscles and joints.

THE GOLDEN RULE

Stretching correctly demands good technique and practice. As in any other discipline, practice makes perfect. Make sure that all your angles are correct as you start the movement. You must move with the right speed and with the right posture. Your focus should be moving the joint as little as possible as you stretch the muscle. Human nature is to take the path of least resistance, which makes us feel flexible and comfortable. However, this approach is not the way to get a good stretch.

CONSIDERATIONS

Should you stretch when warm or cold?

Most people feel more comfortable and flexible when they are warm. However, can you stretch without warming up first? If you follow the basic guidelines on stretching, you will not risk an injury. It can be difficult and impractical to warm up every time if you are trying to correct a condition that requires you to stretch 10 times a day.

Should you stretch before or after a workout?

If you work out to feel good and to stay fit, it is fine to stretch before, after, and even during a workout. If you lift weights, it may help to stretch both the muscle that you are working as well and its antagonist. If the antagonist is flexible and pliable, the stretch will be easier and the risk for injury will decrease. Stretching the calves during a run can help avoid injury, since tight, shortened calf muscles often affecting your stride.

Make it a part of your day

Maximizing the effect of your stretches should be part of your daily habits, just like brushing your teeth or showering. Your muscles need frequent maintenance as well. This is especially true if you suffer from problems related to tight or shortened muscles. Although you might feel silly stretching at work, it can help you avoid getting headaches or throwing your back out. An employer who really cares for his employees will allow for stretching breaks in the morning and afternoon.

What do you need to be able to stretch?

You do not really need any equipment to be able to stretch. All the exercises in this book can be done at home, at work, or at the gym. A wall, a table, a phonebook (to stand on), a towel, or an ironing board all work well as equipment.

The golden rule

Work for the maximum stretch with minimal joint movement.

PERFORMANCE

Several methods for stretching exist, but the basic idea is the same. Stretches should elongate the muscle.

The safest and most effective approach is the PNF (proprioceptive muscular facilitation) method, also called contract-release. This method is based on tricking the body's own defense mechanism. First, stretch the muscle until it starts to work against you, and your body sends a message to the muscle to tighten up and defend itself. As you hold the position, the muscle will dismiss the possibility of danger and the body will relax again.

You can also voluntarily tighten the muscle to calm the body's defenses. The PNF method is designed to make sure that your body does not fight the stretch. Adhere to the four basic principles for the greatest benefit.

STEPS OF THE PNF METHOD

The PNF method can be split into six parts:

1. Assume the correct starting position.
2. Stretch until you reach the ending point.
3. Relax.
4. Tighten the muscle without moving it.
5. Relax.
6. Stretch to the new ending point.

Repeat the last four steps three to six times, depending on the exercise and your goals.

Ending Point

An ending point is a position from which the movement stops for any reason. Certain ending points are movable and others are set. Whenever you stretch a muscle, you will reach an ending point sooner or later. You may stop when you feel a sting or pain in the muscle. The movement may also be stopped by soft tissue (muscle and skin) or bony parts running into each other. During the PNF method, an ending point is reached when you feel a light sting in the muscle. If you reach a different kind of ending point, you need to stop the movement to correct your technique or possibly take a break from stretching that muscle. Certain stretches cannot be performed unless other muscles have been stretched first.

Starting Position

Without the correct starting position, whether standing, sitting, or lying down, it is impossible to stretch effectively. For this reason, you need to spend time learning this position before moving on to the rest of the stretch. If the starting position for a stretch is difficult, you might want to use a mirror or have somebody check your posture. Read the instructions and look at the illustrations carefully before you start.

Stretching

During the stretching phase, you try to elongate the muscle until you feel a light sting. Naturally, the stretch should be done slowly and with control in the right direction to be effective (to prevent activating the body's defense systems). The direction for the stretch will be marked with an arrow.

Relaxation

During the relaxation phase, you simply hold the position at the ending point while relaxing the muscle as much as you can. At this point, you are trying to reduce the body's attempt to tighten the muscle. If you are actively able to relax, the stretch will be more effective.

Contraction

This is another method for distracting the body in order to fool its defenses. You will contract the muscle being stretched against some form of resistance (your own hand, the floor, or the wall) in order to prevent movement. Contracting without moving further disarms the body's defense system. During this phase, the light sting you felt in the previous phase should diminish or disappear. If the pain increases instead, you went too far in the initial stretching phase. If you did everything right, you will now feel able to stretch again until you reach a new ending point.

WHEN TO AVOID STRETCHING

It is almost always beneficial to stretch, but in certain conditions, you might have to take special care or avoid stretching completely.

AGE

Children are naturally more flexible than adults. As we get older, the body becomes stiffer, less pliable, and less adaptable. However, this does not mean that you should stop stretching as you get older. You can always improve your mobility, and you can retain your flexibility by stretching, thereby avoiding some of the aches caused by age. You don't have to be able to do the splits, just to move enough that your muscles can relax. This helps your whole body stay in tune. The most important thing to remember as you get older is to never force a stretch. Also, do not assume that you will achieve results as quickly and easily as you did when you were younger.

AFTER INJURY

After certain injuries, you can start stretching right away. With others, it can be beneficial to wait. In general, you should wait 48 hours after pulling a muscle or getting a Charlie horse before stretching again. If the injury is severe, you might have to wait even longer. If the injury is to a joint, such as a twisted ankle or knee, you should wait to start stretching until the injury has been evaluated. To be sure, contact a naprapath (specialist of neuromusculoskeletal conditions) or physical therapist for an evaluation.

With other acute injuries or conditions, such as a stiff neck or back pain, it is almost always a good idea to start stretching certain muscles. Movement is often the best treatment for this kind of injury. Make sure that you use the correct technique.

Stretching is also recommended for injuries that are caused by repeated movements. These lead to shortened or tightened muscles, which in turn can affect the

tendons. Remember to follow the four basic principles and to stop if the pain increases when you either stretch or contract the muscles.

Kink in the Neck or Back

No exact diagnosis exists for when you throw your back out or get a stiff neck. These afflictions can be a result of anything from muscles cramps and spasms to joints in the spine that lock up (or a combination of these). Any condition that causes pain and decreases mobility needs to be correctly diagnosed so that you can get the right treatment. Doctors often refer to acute backache as the injury, but this diagnosis does nothing to indicate the pain's specific location or cause.

For a long time, doctors routinely prescribed two weeks of bed rest for acute backache. Nowadays, we know that you need to keep moving to heal. Anyone who experiences acute backache should see a naprapath, chiropractor, physical therapist, or doctor for an evaluation.

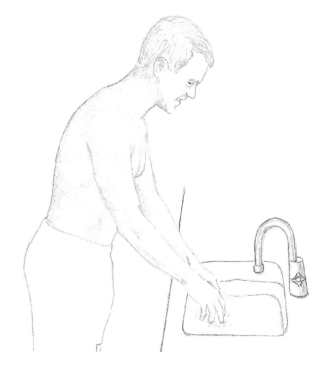

The slight forward lean involved in doing the dishes can cause back problems.

HYPERMOBILITY

Hypermobility refers to joint mobility that is too great. Gymnasts, dancers, or students of the martial arts may experience this. Hypermobility can also be caused by genetic problems. If the mobility of a joint becomes too great, it can injure the joint. The joint and the surrounding ligaments may also start to transmit pain signals.

An interesting phenomenon is that a joint can be extremely mobile even if the muscles surrounding the joint are shortened. So, hypermobility does not necessarily mean that your muscles are relaxed and flexible. To avoid further problems with the joint, you must follow the basic principles of stretching. Technique and the choice of which muscles to stretch determine whether a hypermobile person should stretch. You must know what to stretch and how a healthy stretch should feel.

PREGNANCY

Many women experience pain in the lower back during pregnancy. This comes primarily from the added weight of the fetus, but the muscles also shorten due to their increased workload. Almost all the women whom I have assisted with stretching exercises have felt some pain relief.

If you can stretch without creating pain in the pelvis during or after the stretch, you can continue stretching during pregnancy. Directly after pregnancy, you should allow the ligaments in the pelvic floor to pull together again. You can usually return to a full stretching program 12 weeks after the delivery. Ask a naprapath or a physical therapist if you are unsure how to approach stretching during your pregnancy.

MEDICAL CONSIDERATIONS

No pharmaceuticals or diseases exist that could make stretching negatively affect the body. However, if you have received large quantities of cortisone, you should be more careful than normal. If you have been injected with cortisone, avoid stretching that particular area for the next 10 days. Ask your doctor or health care professional if you are unsure.

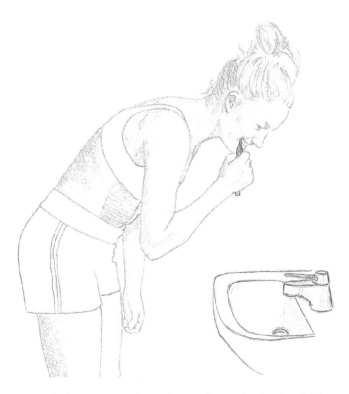

Many daily activities place demands on the back, which can lead to problems. Leaning forward slightly is never a good position for your back.

EXERCISES TO AVOID

In general, all exercises that bring about maximum movement in the joint but do not achieve a stretch in the muscle are not very good. An example of this is the exercise in which you try to stretch the front of your thigh by bringing your heel backward toward your buttocks. In this case, the knee joint is significantly bent, but the muscle in question is not being stretched very much. Part of the movement also adds stress to the lower back. The main problem here lies in the starting position. Instead, try the supine exercise for the rectus femoris on page 86. You will feel a difference in your flexibility.

Avoid the following exercises:

- Stretching the back of the thigh from a standing position
- Stretching the inside of the thigh from a standing position
- Stretching the front of the thigh from a prone position while the calf touches the thigh
- Stretching the gluteal muscles from a seated position
- Stretching the hip flexors from a standing position with a straight back leg
- Stretching the chest with a straight arm below the height of the shoulder
- Stretching the front of the thighs from a kneeling position
- Stretching the front of the thigh from a standing position
- Stretching the muscles between the shoulder blades from a standing position with the upper back rounded and the hands crossed between the knees

Never stretch in the following conditions:

- After a fracture
- During high fever
- When a joint is inflamed
- When open sores or stitches on the skin cover the muscle

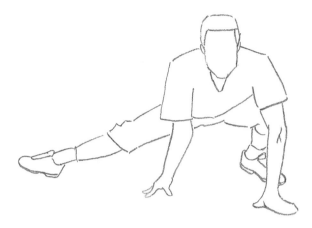

Stretching the inside of the thigh while standing (often called a split) is not recommended. This exercise puts stress on the inside of the knee.

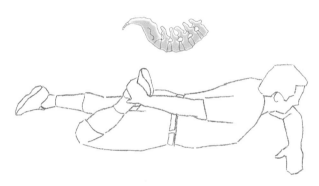

Stretching the front of the thigh while lying down creates a lot of movement in the lower back. It also maximizes the movement of the knee joint.

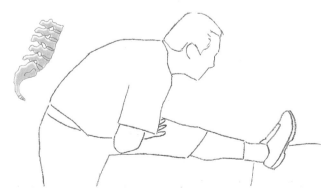

Stretching the back of the thigh with a rounded back and a hyperextended leg puts undue stress on both the knee joint and the back.

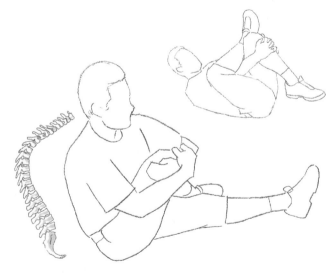

When stretching the gluteal muscles, your lower back should be arched, not rounded as in this picture.

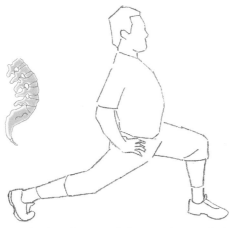

Stretching the hip flexors while standing with the back leg straight is not recommended. When stretching the hip flexors, you should not increase the arch in the lower back. Instead, flatten your back.

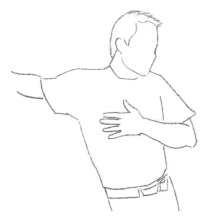

Stretching the chest muscles with a straight arm below the height of the shoulder is not recommended. Keeping the arm straight puts undue stress on the elbow.

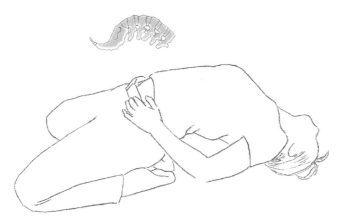

Stretching the front of the thighs from a kneeling position is not recommended, since you end up increasing the arch in the lower back and maximizing the movement in the knee joint.

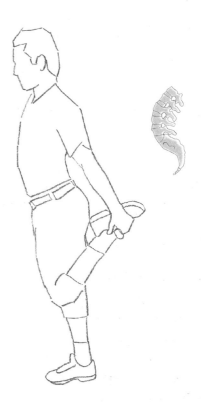

When stretching the front of the thigh while standing, a big part of the movement occurs in the lower back. You also maximize the movement of the knee joint.

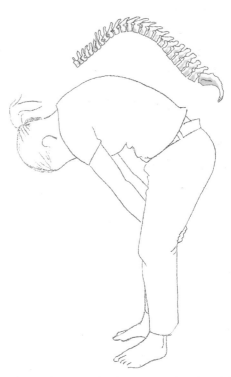

Stretching the muscles between the shoulder blades while standing puts too much stress on the discs in the spine.

GOOD POSTURE HELPS THE BODY

Good posture is kind to the muscles by eliminating unnecessary static work. When the muscles are forced to work statically, they use more energy, thereby generating more lactic acid and creating fatigue. Good posture puts the load as close to the center of the body as possible, making sitting and standing very efficient.

Bad posture can be caused by the following:
- Shortened muscles
- Weak muscles
- Old untreated injuries
- Posture of the people around you (children copy the adults)
- Worries and stress
- Pain

SPINAL COLUMN

The spinal column is the main building block for achieving good posture without excess load. The spinal column and the muscles surrounding it offer the opportunity to treat the body in a beneficial manner.

The spinal column consists of 24 separate vertebrae that are all a little smaller at the top than at the bottom. They are bound together by different joints and ligaments. The sacrum and the tailbone are located at the bottom of the spine. The sacrum is made up of five vertebrae that are fused together into one bone that is wedged between the hip bones. The bone underneath the sacrum is often called the tailbone. It also consists of four or five little vertebrae that are fused together.

The entire spine is covered by a multitude of small muscles. With the exception of the top of the spine, there is a disc between each set of vertebrae.

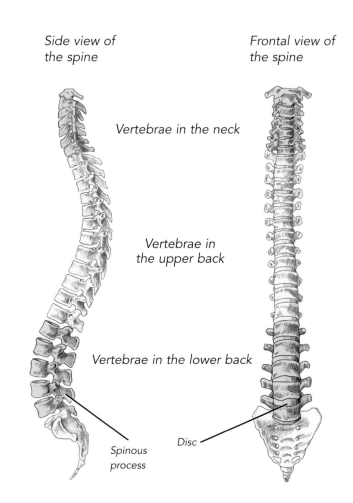

Side view of the spine

Frontal view of the spine

Vertebrae in the neck

Vertebrae in the upper back

Vertebrae in the lower back

Spinous process

Disc

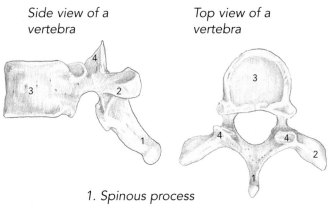

Side view of a vertebra

Top view of a vertebra

1. Spinous process
2. Transverse process
3. Vertebral body
4. Articulations of the spine

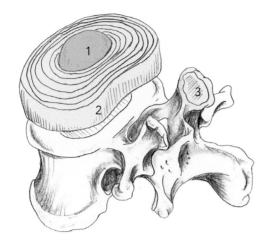

1. Nucleus pulposus = Jellylike substance
2. Annulus fibrosus = Ring of fibrocartilage
3. Articulations of the spine

Movements of the spine include the following:
1. Bending to the side
2. Bending backward
3. Bending forward

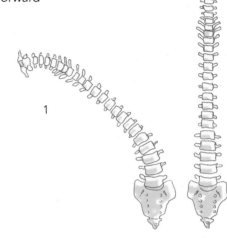

It is made up of a ring of cartilage and a nucleus of a jellylike substance. The discs serve the same purpose of cushioning as the sole of a running shoe does.

They are a buffer that absorbs forces and vibrations. If not for the discs, the vertebrae would get crushed from repeatedly being forced together during standing or walking. The spine is a movable pillar in the center of the body that contains three distinct curves when viewed from the side.

The seven vertebrae of the neck are positioned into an arch, or lordosis. The next twelve in the chest form a rounded shape, or kyphosis. The last five in the lower back create another arch. This shape helps the back absorb force, since it can increase or decrease these curves to relieve pressure. To keep all these movable pieces in place, the spine is covered with ligaments and small muscles that work together to stabilize the back and enable movement.

The spine is subjected to great demands. It is not just there to protect the spinal cord running through it and to keep the body erect. It should also be flexible enough to bend, to absorb forces when we run or walk, and to withstand enormous forces of compression when we lift something heavy. At the same time, it needs to be able to move in several directions. These are the reasons for this ingeniously constructed part of the body.

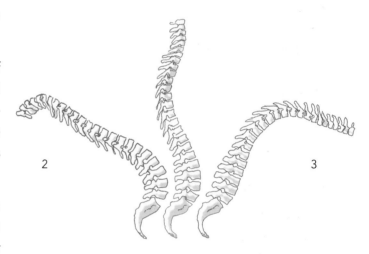

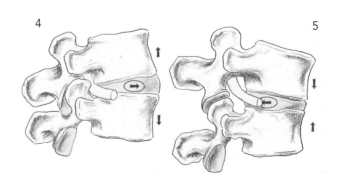

4. Bending backward lessens the space for the nerve.
5. Bending forward increases the space for the nerve but also increases pressure on the front of the disc and forces the nucleus pulposus backward.

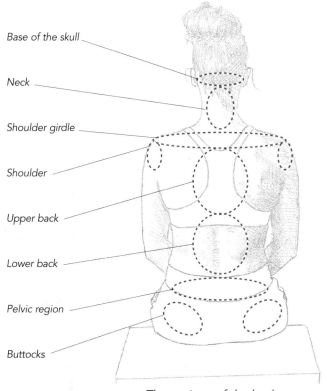

Base of the skull

Neck

Shoulder girdle

Shoulder

Upper back

Lower back

Pelvic region

Buttocks

The regions of the back.

If you really want to rupture a disc, remember to practice these bad habits.

Walk around with bad posture and slouch as much as possible, both when standing and when sitting. If the force from the ground cannot travel through the center of the spine, the damaging leverage on the discs increases up to nine times.

Never use your legs when lifting heavy things. Lifting with straight legs and a bent back are ideal ways to rupture a disc, whether during a single incident or over time. If you attempt to turn your body while lifting, you increase your chances of disc injury by several percent.

It might be enough to just sit a lot, day in and day out over the years. Persistence is rewarded.

Remember that things do not happen by themselves.

RUPTURED DISCS

When a disc is ruptured, the cartilage ring breaks, and the jellylike center leaks out. If you are unlucky, this rupture will put pressure on a nerve, creating irritation and inflammation that generates pain. The pain may be local or may radiate to the area that the pinched nerve controls through impulses. The most common area for rupture is between the fourth and fifth lumbar vertebrae in the lower back. Unfortunately, this is also where the sciatic nerve exits the spine. If this nerve is pinched, pain radiates down the leg and into the foot, maybe even diminishing reflexes and motor control. However, most ruptured discs are asymptomatic, which means that they do not elicit any pain or any symptoms. In reality, most people have ruptured at least one disc without knowing it by age 45.

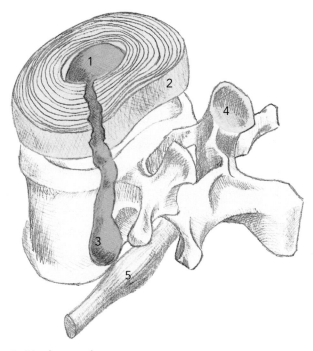

1. *Nucleus pulposus*
2. *Annulus fibrosus*
3. *Nucleus pulposus leaks toward a nerve (item 5)*
4. *Articulations of the spine*

ABDOMINAL MUSCLES

The problem with the abs is that we know where they are and how to train them, but we don't know how to use them when we really need them. The abs play an important role for your posture and the well-being of your spine. They create stability between the upper and lower body and take pressure off the discs in the spine.

The four main muscles that are considered part of the abs are the straight muscle in front, the external and internal obliques, and the transversus abdominis. Their main functions include bending the trunk forward, turning the trunk, and bending the trunk sideways. Although these are all important functions, their most important function is interabdominal pressure. This is created by taking a breath, closing the mouth, and tightening the abdominal muscles. Pressure in the abdominal cavity increases, which separates the vertebrae from each other and decreases the pressure on the discs. Strong interabdominal pressure can decrease the pressure of the bottom disc as much as 50 percent and relieve the disc above it as much as 30 percent. Knowing this, it is easy to understand why you should create this pressure with your abs when lifting both heavy and light loads.

In order to get this decreased pressure, you must be able to tighten your abs. It might sound simple, but a lot of people cannot do this correctly. Some think that the abs are tightened by pushing the belly out, while others try to suck it in. Neither action creates the desired effect.

Test Your Abs

• Stand with your back against a wall. Your heels, buttocks, shoulder blades, and the back of your head should all touch the wall. Now, try to push your lower back into the wall, keeping your butt or shoulders against it. If you cannot figure out if your lower back is actually moving towards the wall, place your hand between the two.

• Lie flat on your back with your legs and feet together. Normally, you be able to feel some space between your lower back and the floor. Now, try to push your back down into the floor. Feel free to keep your hands between your lower back and the floor so that you can appreciate how hard you are able to push your lower back down.

In these exercises, the abs work almost exclusively. Some people cannot make the lower back move toward the wall or the floor at all; they cannot get the abs to fire. They will turn and twist the body without moving the lower back any closer to the goal. Work on successfully doing this test. It will help you use and rely on your abs, thereby helping you create posture that is better and more relaxed.

If tightening your abs seems impossible, try coughing or bearing down. You might also find it difficult to tighten your abs if other muscles are too tight or are shortened, such as the hip flexors or the quads on the front of your legs. Stretches for these muscles are described on pages 83 and 86 in the exercise section of the book.

GOOD POSTURE

STANDING

When viewed from the side, your ear, shoulder, hip, knee, and foot should all be in line with each other, forming the plumb line of the body. When the spine assumes its normal curvature, the forces absorbed by the spine can travel straight through each vertebra and disc. Your knees should be slightly bent rather than hyperextended.

Common Mistakes

- Pushing the chin forward so that the ear is in front of the shoulder, creating the neck position of a vulture
- Rounding the shoulders forward, creating a hump back in the upper back
- Pushing the hips forward and significantly arching the lower back (regrettably a resting position for many)
- Tilting the hips backward, eliminating the arch of the lower back and creating something I call *taxicab ass*

When viewed from the front, the head should be straight and not tilted or rotated. (This distinction is sometimes difficult to see since it can be very minute.) The shoulders should be lowered and level with one another. The feet should be placed hip-width apart, and the toes should point out slightly.

This might seem very simple at first. However, if you look around you will find that very few people actually stand like this. They lean forward, backward, or to the side. They may also bear more weight on one leg than on the other.

This is how to stand correctly:

- The feet should be hip-width apart with the toes pointing out a couple of degrees
- Weight should be equally borne on both the heel and the ball of the foot.
- The knees should be slightly bent. First, try hyperextending the knees and then bending them slightly. It is enough to bring the knees forward about 1 inch (2.5 cm).
- The abs should be slightly tightened to create stability.
- The spine should have its natural curves.
- The shoulders should be lowered.
- The head should be straight.

You can test your posture by having somebody push down on your shoulders. If you are standing correctly, you will not sway. It is especially important that the abdomen is not pushed forward by this pressure. If it is, the arch in the lower back is too great. You can correct this by tightening up your abs and flattening your lower back, just as you did in the exercise against the wall.

GOOD POSTURE

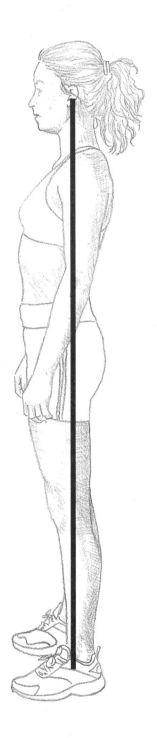

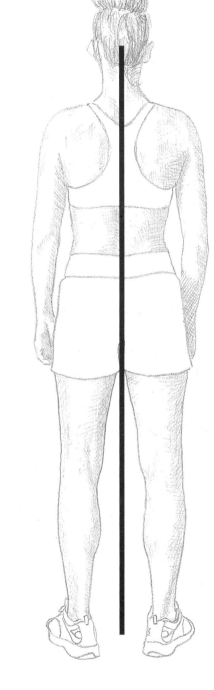

The plumb line is an imaginary line running through the ear, shoulder, spine, knee, and the outside of the ankle.

The weight of the body should be evenly distributed across the left and right sides of this line.

BAD POSTURE

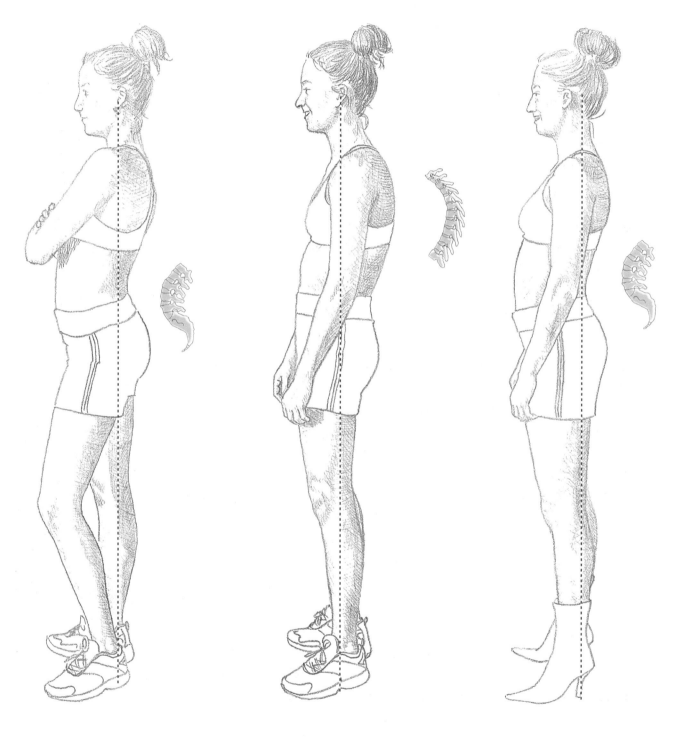

Leaning on one leg and arching the back moves the plumb line too far back.

Hunching over moves the plumb line too far forward.

Wearing high heels tends to move the plumb line too far back.

SITTING

Even if it is not recommended, sometimes you must sit down. When you sit, it is crucial that you remain very active. Do not relax all your muscles or slouch. Instead, keep certain muscles active. In most cases, it is difficult to sit correctly for a long period of time. However, this gives you a reason to get up and move around for a while.

Sitting correctly does not necessarily require a good chair, but it does require that you know how to stand correctly. If you know how to stand correctly, you will also be aware of whether the spine is in the correct position when you are sitting. Even when you sit, the curvature of your back still determines the effect of the load on the rest of your body.

Remember to sit with your feet planted wide apart on the floor for good support. If you sit on a taller chair, it is easier to get a greater angle between your thighs and your back. This angle should be at least 45 degrees. Your back should be straight to maintain the same curvature as when you are standing. Keep your shoulders lowered and in line with your ears. Avoid using a backrest as much as possible. Sitting actively is the best way to protect the back. Using a backrest inevitably decreases the natural arch of the back, which places more pressure on the spinal discs. On top of that, you are no longer using the muscles to keep yourself upright. Instead, you rely on passive structures, such as ligaments and joint capsules, to stay up.

Occasionally sitting down can be good if you have not practiced standing properly often enough. However, a good and expensive chair is no guarantee for a pain-free and healthy back. It all depends on how long you sit, how you sit, and how strong and flexible your muscles are.

Always remember that there is a difference between just sitting and working while sitting when you buy a chair.

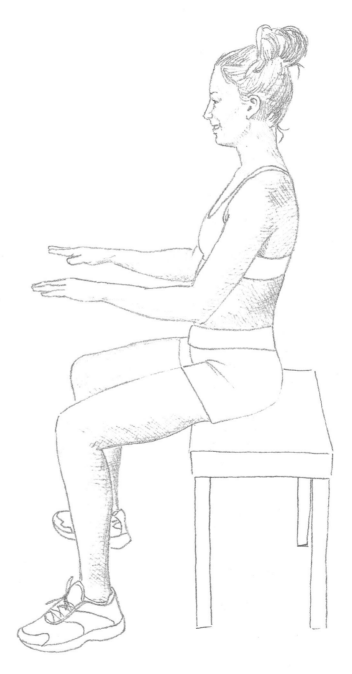

The spine should have the same curvature when you are seated as when you are standing with good posture.

Consequences of Poor Posture

If you sit a lot or are inactive, you will lose the ability to stand correctly. You might even have a hard time walking or running because the important muscles for these functions become tight and shortened when you sit.

Poor posture can lead to the following conditions:

- Shortened, tight muscles continue to worsen posture.
- Poor movement pattern when running or walking can cause other injuries.
- Trigger points in the muscles can cause local discomfort or radiating pain in the arms and legs.
- Headaches cause tension and increase lactic acid in the muscles, making the headache even worse.

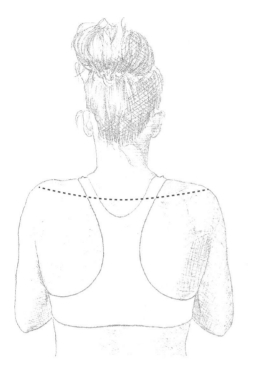

When you are stressed, the shoulders have a tendency to lift, which makes the muscles work statically.

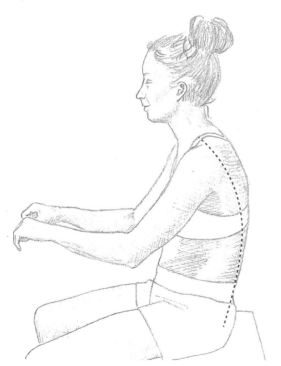

A hunched posture while sitting increases the pressure on the discs in the lower back as much as tenfold. Even the muscles in the neck must work statically to keep the head from falling forward.

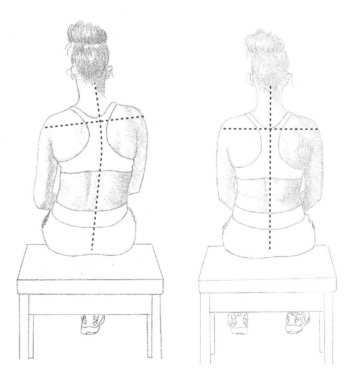

Crossing your legs while sitting pushes the body in one direction. The other muscles have to compensate so you don't fall sideways.

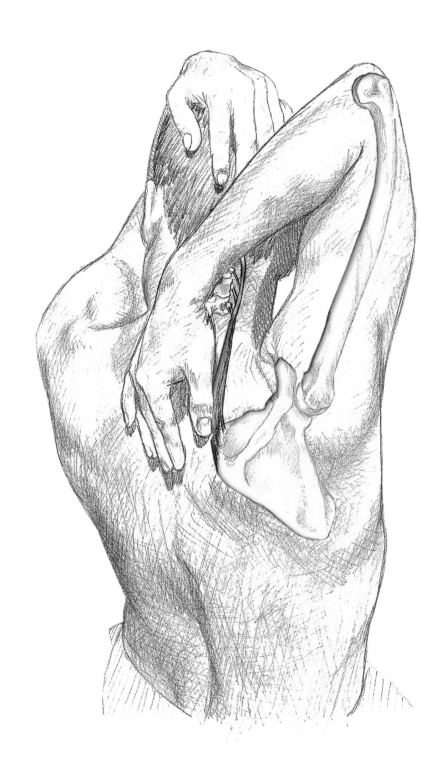

TARGETED STRETCHES

UPPER TRAPEZIUS

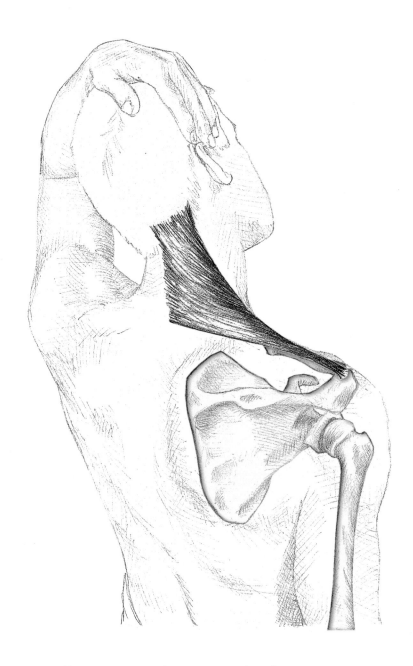

This exercise is very effective when done correctly. The starting position and hand placement are very important; the shoulder must stay down during the stretch in order to decrease the static tension in the muscle. You do not need to go all out when performing this exercise. You can simply do steps 1 and 2.

MUSCLE FACTS

The trapezius is a large, flat muscle close to the skin that covers the shoulder, the neck, and the upper back. The trapezius raises the shoulder, bringing the shoulder blades closer to each other, rotates the head, and helps the head lean to the side.

Causes of Tightness

The muscle can become tight and shortened when you subconsciously lift the shoulder. This causes enduring static tension in the shoulder, leading to general tension in the area. The reason for lifting your shoulder can be anything from being cold to feeling stressed.

It is very common to have difficulty relaxing the neck and shoulders when you feel stressed; this area is where the tension shows up. Since the trapezius raises the shoulder, it follows that if you are often stressed, this muscle never gets to relax. Therefore, it will become very tight and short, leading to pain and fatigue.

Symptoms of Tightness

- Headache at the base of the skull, above the ear, outside of the eye, or behind the eye
- Local pain across the shoulder girdle
- Local pain between the shoulder blades
- Difficulty rotating or tilting your head sideways

Flexibility Test

You should be able to tilt your head approximately 45 degrees to the side and to rotate your head about 90 degrees in each direction.

Precautions

Avoid this exercise if, during a stretch, the pain is concentrated under the ear instead of throughout the muscle.

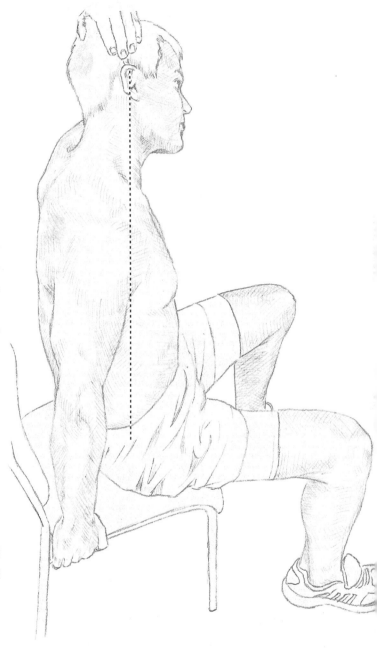

Make sure that your head is in line with your upper body.

TECHNIQUE

Sit·on a chair or bench with your feet wide apart and your back and abs slightly tightened. Reach behind you with your right hand and grab the edge of the chair. Lean your upper body to the left, keeping your head upright. You will feel a light pull in your right shoulder or your upper arm.

Next, try to lift your right shoulder toward the ceiling for five seconds. Do not allow your body to move sideways. Relax for a couple of seconds and then lean your upper body a little more to the side. You have now reached the correct starting position for the stretch.

Carefully lean your head to the left side and rotate it slightly to the right. Put your left hand against your head and stretch the muscle for 5 to 10 seconds by carefully pulling your head to the side. Stop the movement when you feel a slight sting in your neck and shoulder. Allow the muscle to relax for 5 to 10 seconds.

Deepen the stretch by moving the head to the left until you reach a new ending point.

Repeat two or three times.

Common Mistakes
• Failing to sit up straight
• Leaning the head forward
• Placing the hand on the chair too far forward

Comments
If you find it difficult to get a good stretch in the muscle, you might want to try some deep-tissue massage to relax the muscle and make it more receptive to stretching. Don't rush the exercise. Instead, take your time in the beginning.

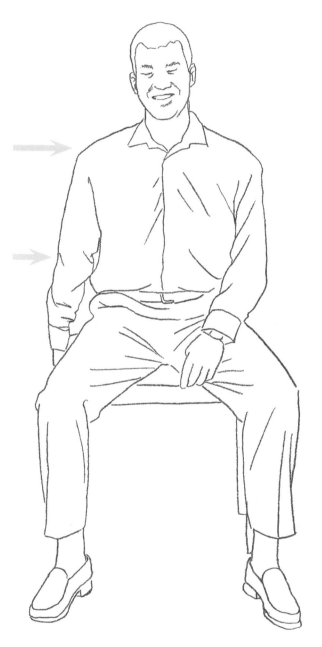

Assume the starting position with your hand placed behind you diagonally. Lean your upper body to the side to lower your shoulder.

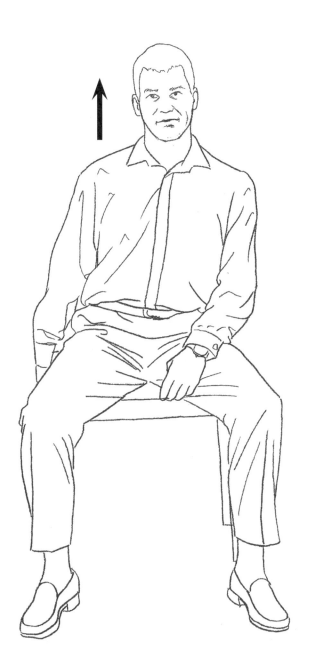

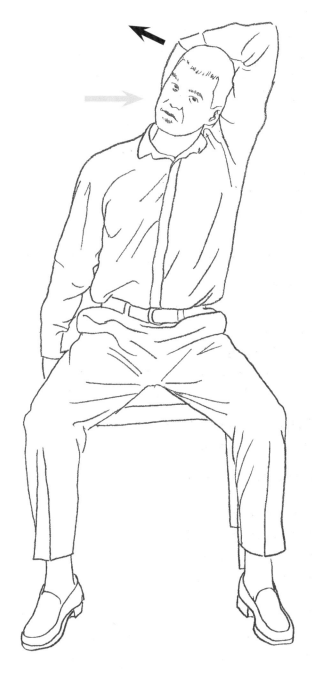

Resist by raising your shoulder toward the ceiling. Next, relax your shoulder and lean to the side more.

Stretch by carefully moving your head sideways while slightly rotating it in the opposite direction. Resist by carefully pushing your head into your hand.

STERNOCLEIDOMASTOID

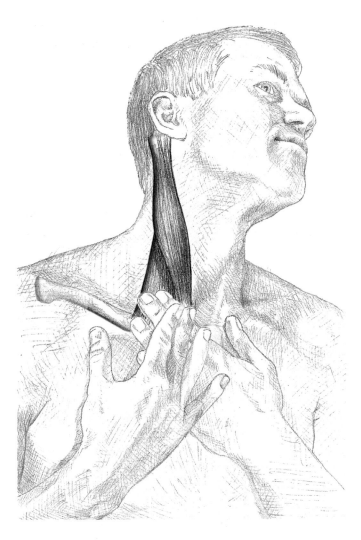

This exercise can feel a little awkward because the muscle is in a sensitive location. Avoid the exercise if it is too uncomfortable. In the beginning, you might want to have a therapist help you with it. To easily locate the muscle, stand in front of a mirror and turn your head to one side. This should cause the muscle to appear clearly.

MUSCLE FACTS

This round muscle, close to the skin at the front of the neck, is easy to see. It runs from the inside of the clavicle along the side of the neck, attaching to the base of the skull just behind the ear. The sternocleidomastoid leans and rotates the head to the side. It also assists in forceful inhalation and tilts the bottom of the neck forward and the head backward.

Causes of Tightness

Bad posture, such as sitting hunched over and looking at a television or computer screen, can cause this muscle to shorten. Bad posture can also result from a shortened pectoralis major. The posture created by a shortened sternocleidomastoid is sometimes called vulture neck, since the profile is reminiscent of a how a vulture carries its neck and head.

Since people under stress often breathe forcefully and raise their shoulders, this muscle can be forced to work statically for long periods of time, leading to tension and pain.

Symptoms of Tightness
• Headache at the top of the head
• Problems aligning the head straight above the spine

Flexibility Test

Stand with your back and the back of your head against a wall. Put one of your hands behind your neck and try to push your neck toward the wall. You should be able to push it against your hand.

Precautions

Avoid this exercise if it causes pain in your neck, dizziness, or difficulty breathing.

TECHNIQUE

This exercise can be done either while sitting or while standing.

Find the muscle's attachment point on the right side of the clavicle, and then place three fingers of your right hand over the bottom inch (2.5 cm) of the muscle. Put your left hand on top of your fingers and keep it there.

Move your head slightly backward and to the left until you feel a slight burn on the right side of your neck. Next, relax the muscle for 5 to 10 seconds.

Resist by moving your head back toward the starting position. You can slow the movement by putting one hand on your forehead and pushing your head into your hand for 5 to 10 seconds. Relax the muscle for 5 to 10 seconds.

Deepen the stretch by bringing your head backward and to the side until you reach a new ending point.

Repeat two or three times.

Common Mistakes
- Incorrect muscle placement
- Rotating the head in the wrong direction

Comments

If you have difficulty with this exercise, bring your head forward before positioning the muscle to achieve a stretch more quickly.

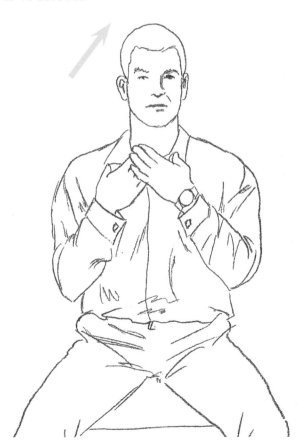

Position the muscles using your fingers. Lean your head back and to the side.

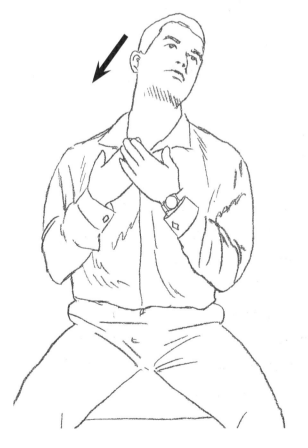

Resist by moving your head back toward the starting position.

SCALENES

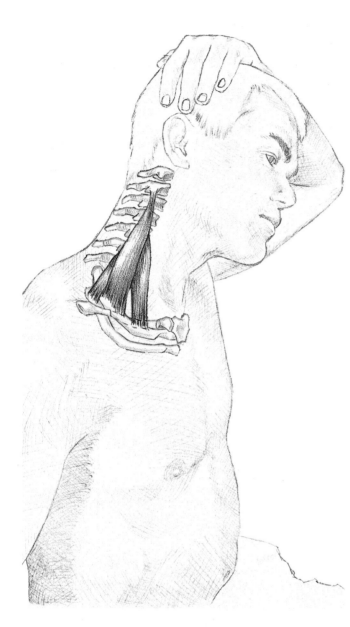

This exercise is similar to that for the upper trapezius on page 26. The difference is that the head is tilted straight to one side without rotation.

MUSCLE FACTS

The scalene muscles are situated on the side of the neck between the upper part of the trapezius and the sterno-cleidomastoid. They run between the cervical vertebrae and the two top ribs. The scalenes help the head lean to the side and assist during forced inhalation.

Causes of Tightness

Habitually sitting with your head leaning toward one side (for example, holding the phone between your cheek and shoulder) can cause the scalenes to tighten up and shorten.

These muscles are considered part of the stress muscles, since forced breathing increases during stress.

Symptoms of Tightness

• Difficulty tilting the head to the side
• Numbness or tingling in the hand or arm

Flexibility Test

You should be able to tilt your head about 45 degrees to the side.

Precautions

Avoid this exercise if you have pain in your neck during the stretch.

TECHNIQUE

Sit on a chair or bench with your feet wide apart and your back and abs slightly tightened. Reach behind you with your right hand and grab the edge of the chair. Lean your upper body to the right, keeping your head upright. You will feel a light pull in your right shoulder or your upper arm.

Next, try to lift your right shoulder toward the ceiling for five seconds. Do not let your body move sideways. Relax for a couple of seconds, and then lean your upper body to the side a little more. You have now reached the correct starting position for the stretch.

Carefully lean your head to the left side. Move your left hand over your head and rest it on the right side of your neck. Stretch the muscle for 5 to 10 seconds by carefully pulling your head to the left side. Stop the movement when you feel a slight sting in the right side of your neck. Relax the muscle for 5 to 10 seconds.

Deepen the stretch by pulling your head to the left until you reach a new ending point.

Repeat two or three times.

Common Mistakes
- Failing to sit up straight during the exercise
- Moving the head out of alignment with the spine
- Gripping the head instead of the neck

Comments
If you have difficulty with this exercise, spend some time stretching the trapezius and sternocleidomastoid muscles before trying again.

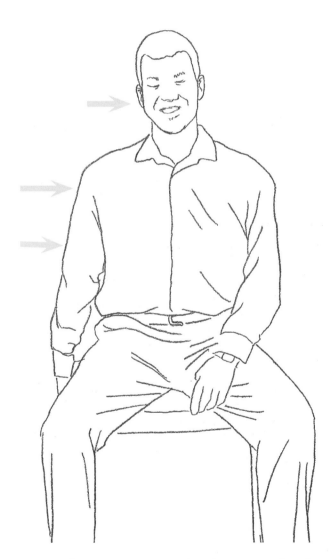

Assume the starting position by placing your hand behind you diagonally. Lean your head and body straight out to the side.

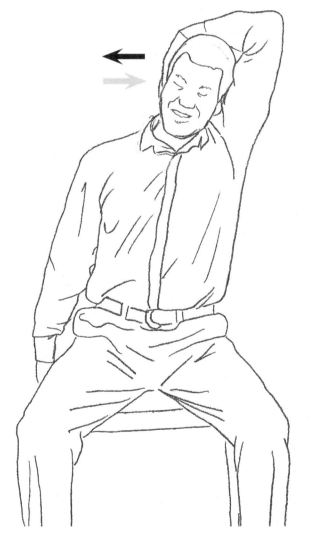

Create resistance by pushing your head against your hand.

SUBOCCIPITALS

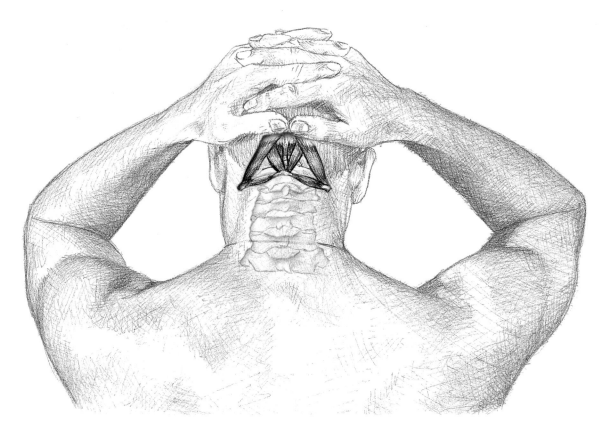

In this exercise, there are two main considerations. Do not let the upper body collapse forward (only the neck should flex forward) and be aware of your thumb placement. For the best results, push your thumbs up into the soft tissue right below the base of your skull.

MUSCLE FACTS

This group of muscles is situated right under the base of the skull. It runs from the top two cervical vertebrae and attaches to the base of the skull. The suboccipital muscles bend the head backward, stabilize the head, and make fine adjustments to the head's movements.

Causes of Tightness

Poor posture that places the head in front of the body makes these muscles work statically to direct your gaze forward instead of at the ground. This process causes them to shorten.

The suboccipital muscles are also activated by stress, especially if you grind your teeth or clench your jaw at night. If you wake up with a headache, you may be overworking these muscles during the night.

Symptoms of Tightness

• Difficulty putting your chin on your chest
• Headache at the bottom of the skull or at the top of the head

Flexibility Test

Since the suboccipital muscles create a movement similar to that of the sternocleidomastoid, you can use the same mobility test. Stiffness usually develops in both muscles at the same time.

Stand with your back and the back of your head against a wall. Put one of your hands behind your neck and try to push your neck toward the wall. You should be able to push your neck against your hand.

Precautions

Avoid this exercise if it causes neck pain or light-headedness.

TECHNIQUE

This exercise can be done either while sitting down or lying on your back. Interlock your fingers and place your hands at the base of your skull. Use your thumbs to push on the muscles right under the base of the skull. Stretch the muscles by slowly pushing your head forward for 5 to 10 seconds. Feel how the muscle pushes against your thumbs. Next, relax the muscles for 5 to 10 seconds.

Deepen the stretch by pushing your head forward until you feel a stretch or light sting in the muscles. This is the new ending point.

Repeat two or three times.

Common Mistakes

• Failing to sit up straight
• Pushing the head down instead of moving it forward

Comments

If you find it difficult to achieve a good stretch, use your thumbs to massage the area below the base of your skull for a couple of minutes or let a therapist assist you until you can do the exercise by yourself.

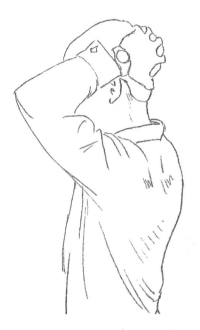

Place your thumbs in the soft tissue directly under the base of your skull. Avoid hunching over as you lean your head forward.

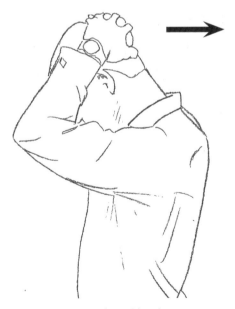

Resist by pressing your head back against your hands.

LEVATOR SCAPULAE (VERSION 1)

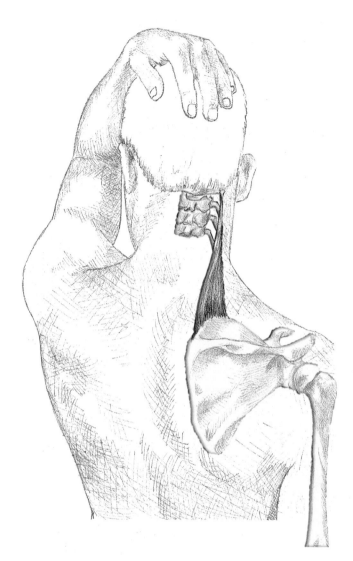

MUSCLE FACTS

The levator scapulae runs between the upper part of the shoulder blades and the top four cervical vertebrae. It is a thin, flat muscle located just below the upper part of the trapezius.

It rotates and tilts the head to the side. When both sides of the muscle work simultaneously, it raises the shoulder girdle and bends the head backward.

Causes of Tightness

The levator scapulae is shortened by bad posture, by permanently raising the shoulder or the shoulder girdle, or by holding a phone between the cheek and the shoulder.

Since the levator scapulae raises the shoulder girdle, it also works statically in times of stress since the shoulders are often raised in response to tension.

Symptoms of Tightness

• Difficulty rotating the head
• Difficulty placing the chin on the chest
• Headache at the back of the head
• Kink in the neck

Flexibility Test

You should be able to rotate the head approximately 90 degrees and to bend the neck approximately 45 degrees to the side.

Precautions

Avoid this exercise if it causes pain in the neck.

TECHNIQUE

Sit on a chair or bench with your feet wide apart and your back and abs slightly tightened. Reach behind you with your right hand and grab the edge of the chair. Lean your upper body to the left, keeping your head upright. You will feel a light pull in your right shoulder or upper arm.

As always, it is important to start in the correct position when stretching. Hunching over while sitting prevents you from stretching as well as you could if you were sitting up straight. Be aware of the rotation of your head. When you have turned your head 45 degrees and you are starting to bend it forward, you must make sure that everything is in line so that you do not pull the muscle at a bad angle.

Now try to lift your right shoulder toward the ceiling for five seconds. Do not allow your body to move sideways. Relax for a couple of seconds and then lean your upper body a little more to the side. You have now reached the correct starting position for the stretch.

Rotate your head 45 degrees to the left. Place your left hand behind your head and gently pull it at an angle toward your knee. Stretch the muscle in this manner for 5 to 10 seconds. Stop the movement when you feel a slight sting in the right side of your neck. Next, relax the muscle for 5 to 10 seconds.

Resist by carefully pushing your head backward into your hand. Next, relax the muscle for 5 to 10 seconds.

Deepen the stretch by slowly pulling your head toward your chest in the direction of your knee until you reach a new ending point.

Repeat two or three times.

Common Mistakes
- Failing to sit up straight
- Compressing the neck instead of moving the head forward and down
- Rotating the head either too much or not enough
- Movement does not follow the direction of the nose straight toward the knee

Comments
This muscle can be hard to stretch if other muscles are tight. If you find this exercise difficult, try to stretch the upper part of the trapezius and the suboccipital muscles first.

In the starting position, place your hand behind you diagonally and rotate your head 45 degrees. Bring your head down toward your left knee without hunching over.

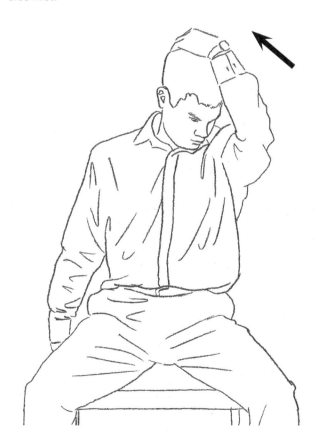

Resist by pressing your head into your hand.

LEVATOR SCAPULAE (VERSION 2)

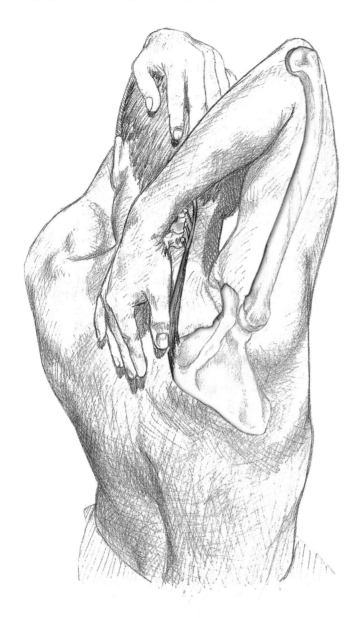

TECHNIQUE

Sit on a chair or bench with your feet wide apart and your back and abs slightly tightened. Bring your right arm over your head, bend your elbow, and place your hand against your neck. Place your left hand behind your head.

Rotate the head 45 degrees to the left so that your nose points toward your left knee. Use your left hand to gently pull your head toward your left knee at an angle until you feel a slight sting in the right side of your neck. Stretch in this manner for 5 to 10 seconds. Next, relax the muscle for 5 to 10 seconds.

Resist by carefully pushing your head back toward your left hand. Next, relax the muscle for 5 to 10 seconds.

Deepen the stretch by continuing to pull the head toward the knee until you reach a new ending point.

Repeat two or three times.

Common Mistakes
- Failing to sit up straight
- Compressing the neck instead of moving the head forward and down
- Rotating the head either too much or not enough
- Movement does not follow the direction of the nose straight toward the knee

Comments
It can be difficult to stretch this muscle well if your shoulder joint is tight. If you have this problem, try stretching the latissimus dorsi and pectoralis major first.

This version is similar to the previous exercise for this muscle. The head position, movement, and direction are identical. However, in this version, you will try to increase the stretch by rotating your shoulder blade externally as you bring your arm above your head.

Precautions
Avoid this exercise if you have pain in the shoulder joint or neck.

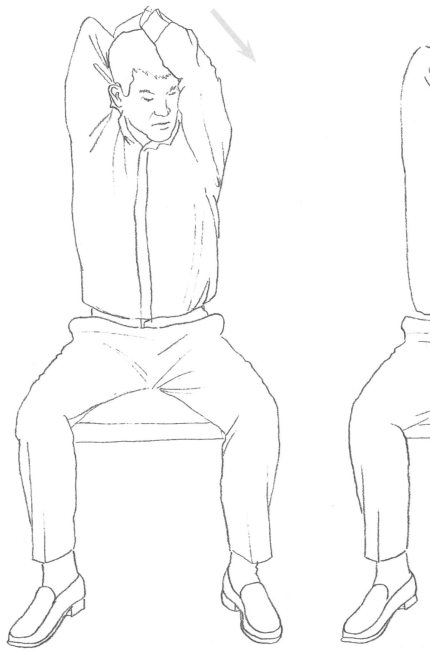

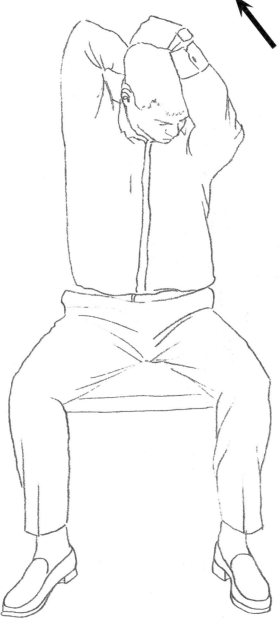

Draw your arm behind your neck as far as you can. Bring your head forward and to the side in the direction of your left knee.

Resist by pressing your head back into your hand.

PECTORALIS MAJOR (VERSION 1)

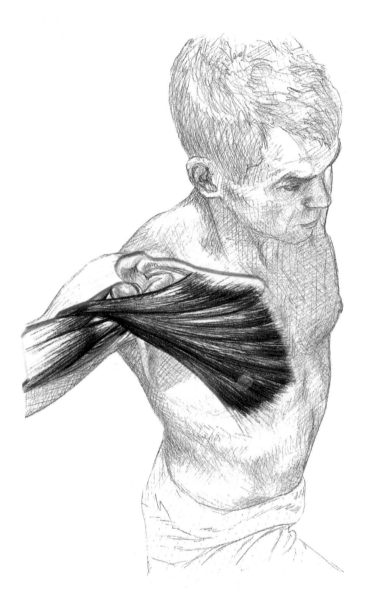

Hypermobility in the shoulder joint where most of the movement takes place can make the pectoralis major difficult to stretch. It can also be difficult to stretch if the muscle is too tight. Technique is very important in this exercise. Keep the abs tight to prevent arching the lower back.

MUSCLE FACTS

The pectoralis major is a large muscle located near the skin in front of the rib cage. It originates in the area near the clavicle, the sternum, and the top of the abs. From there, it runs toward the upper arm. The pectoralis major rotates the arm internally and moves the shoulder blade forward.

Causes of Tightness

The pectoralis major is shortened by bad posture habits, such as hunching over or working with your arms extended in front of you. Hair dressers, massage therapists, and people who work with computers are often affected.

The pectoralis major is not considered to be directly affected by stress, but some people feel relaxed after stretching it. Some even find it easier to breathe. Reduced tension in the pectoralis major often leads to better posture, which allows other muscles to relax as well.

Symptoms of Tightness

- Vulture-neck posture (head juts out in front of the body)
- Pain or muscle spasms between the shoulder blades
- Pain across the sternum
- Pressure across the chest (similar to angina)
- Sensations of tingling and numbness in the arms, especially at night

Flexibility Test

Test 1

Stand with your back against a wall. Move both arms straight out to the side until your elbows are slightly above your shoulders. Bend your arms to 90 degrees and turn them so that your forearms are flat against the wall and your upper arms are level with your shoulders. You should be able to touch your entire forearm and back of your hand to the wall without arching your lower back.

Test 2

Stand facing a right-angled corner. Place one foot in the corner and bend your arms to 90 degrees. Next, place your elbows against the walls and turn them so that your forearms are flat against the wall and your upper arms are level with your shoulders. Lean your upper body into the corner. If you are really flexible, your chest will move closer to the corner.

Precautions

Avoid this exercise if you have pain in your shoulder joint, between your shoulder blades, or in your lower back during the stretch.

TECHNIQUE

Stand with your right hand and forearm positioned against a door frame. Make sure that the elbow is placed a little higher than the shoulder is. Tighten up your abs to prevent arching the lower back. Take one step forward with your right foot.

Stretch for 5 to 10 seconds by slowly bending your right leg. This causes your body to lean forward and down. Stop the movement when you feel a slight sting across the chest muscle. Next, relax the muscle for 5 to 10 seconds.

Resist by pressing your right elbow against the door frame for 5 to 10 seconds. Next, relax for 5 to 10 seconds.

Repeat two or three times.

Common Mistakes

• Positioning the elbow too low
• Failing to tighten the abs (therefore arching the lower back)

Comments

It can be difficult to achieve a good stretch in the muscle if you already have a lot of mobility in your shoulder joint. If so, raise your arm a bit higher.

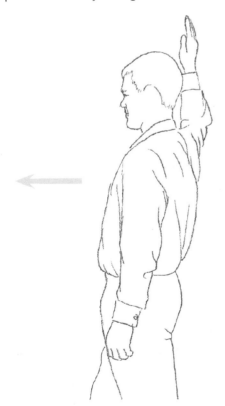

Keep your elbow slightly higher than your shoulder. Tighten your abs and lean your upper body forward.

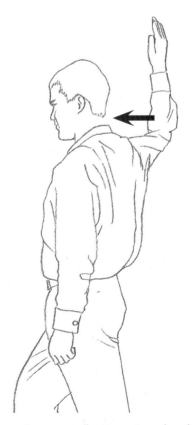

Resist by pressing your elbow against the door frame without actually moving your body.

PECTORALIS MAJOR (VERSION 2)

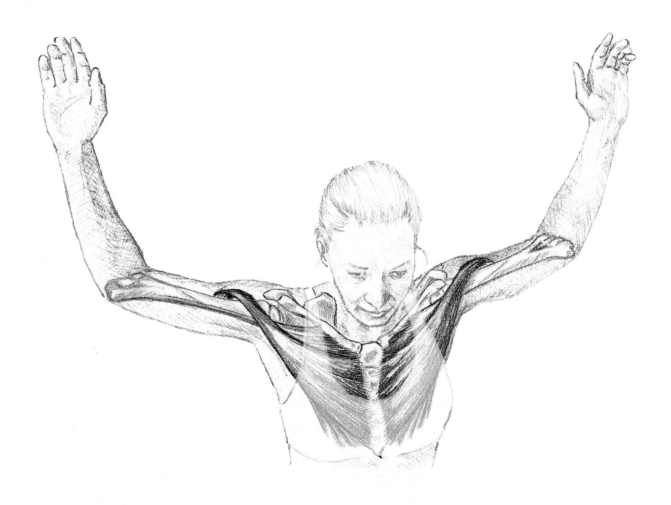

This exercise is very effective if you would like to become flexible in the pecs, the muscles surrounding the ribs, and those between the ribs and the spine. This exercise stretches both sides of the chest muscle at the same time. Therefore, be careful to place both elbows at the same height so that you stretch both sides equally. You should also remember to alternate the position of the front leg.

TECHNIQUE

Stand facing a right-angled corner. Place one foot in the corner and your hands and forearms against the walls. Your elbows should be positioned slightly higher than your shoulder blades, and your forearms should point toward the ceiling. Tighten up the abs to prevent arching your lower back.

Stretch for 5 to 10 seconds by bending the front leg and leaning your body into the corner until you feel a light sting or stretch in the chest muscle. Next, relax the muscle for 5 to 10 seconds.

Resist by pressing both elbows into the walls, keeping the upper body still. The stinging feeling in the muscle should subside. Relax the muscle for 5 to 10 seconds.

Deepen the stretch by bending your leg and leaning your upper body into the corner until you feel the slight sting again. This is your new ending point.

Repeat two or three times.

Common Mistakes
- Keeping the elbows too low
- Pointing the forearms in rather than straight up
- Failing to tighten the abs, allowing the lower back to arch

Comments

If you are very inflexible and have difficulty achieving a stretch, try version 1 for a while before attempting this exercise. Massaging the muscle may also help it relax.

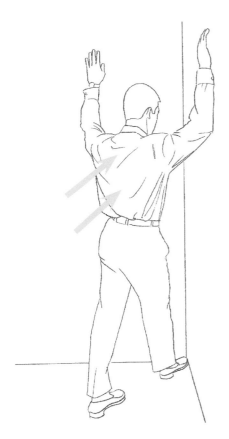

Keep both elbows slightly above your shoulders. Tighten your abs and lean your upper body into the corner.

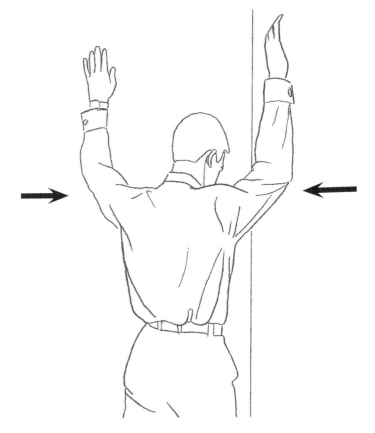

Resist by pressing your elbows against the wall without actually moving your body.

PECTORALIS MINOR (STANDING VERSION)

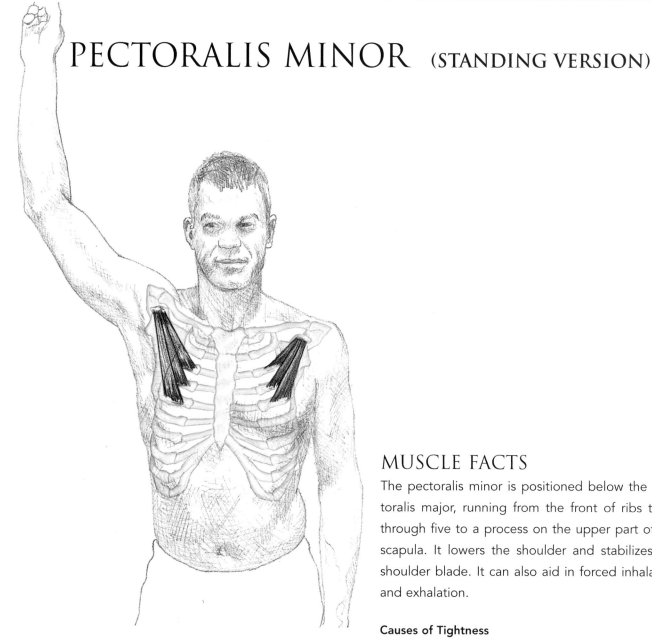

It can be tough to get a good stretch in the pectoralis minor that you can really feel, since the muscle can be very tight and the movement it makes can be small. Even if you do not feel very much, the stretch will still do you good. This stretch provides relief for numbness in the hands and arms at night. You will know this muscle is working if you feel something in your arm or hand while stretching. Don't be concerned; this feeling will subside as your muscles become more flexible.

MUSCLE FACTS

The pectoralis minor is positioned below the pectoralis major, running from the front of ribs three through five to a process on the upper part of the scapula. It lowers the shoulder and stabilizes the shoulder blade. It can also aid in forced inhalation and exhalation.

Causes of Tightness

Prolonged static work and bad posture can cause this muscle to tighten up. As with other muscles, stress increases tension in the upper chest, especially if breathing becomes more rapid.

Symptoms of Tightness

- Numbness and pain radiating into the arm
- Symptoms similar to tennis elbow
- Difficulty inhaling deeply
- Pain across the muscle (similar to symptoms of angina or heart attack)

Precautions

Avoid this exercise if you have pain in the shoulder joint or neck while stretching.

TECHNIQUE

Stand with your right forearm and hand against a door frame. Position your elbow considerably higher than your shoulder joint. Your forearm should face straight up, forming a 130-degree angle between your body and your elbow. Tighten up your abs to prevent arching your lower back. Take one step forward with your right foot.

Stretch for 5 to 10 seconds by slowly bending the right leg, causing your upper body to slowly lean forward and down. Stop the movement when you feel a slight sting in the muscle. Relax the muscle for 5 to 10 seconds.

Resist by slowly pushing your right elbow forward for 5 to 10 seconds. Relax for 5 to 10 seconds.

Deepen the stretch by bending the right leg until you feel a slight sting. This is your new ending point.

Repeat two or three times.

Common Mistakes
- Positioning the elbow either too high or too low
- Lack of flexibility in the shoulder joint
- Failing to tighten the muscle enough, causing an arch in the back

Comments

This is a difficult exercise because the muscle can be hard to reach. Try stretching the pectoralis major before working the pectoralis minor.

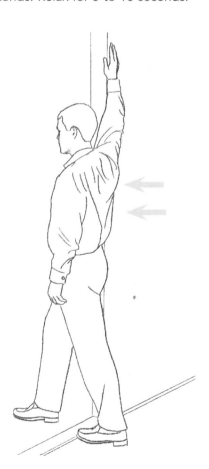

Be sure to keep your elbow at eye height. Tighten your abs and lean your upper body forward.

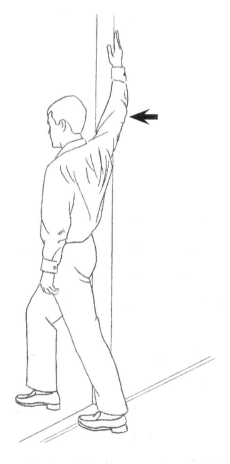

Resist by pressing your elbow against the door frame without actually moving your body.

45

PECTORALIS MINOR (SEATED VERSION)

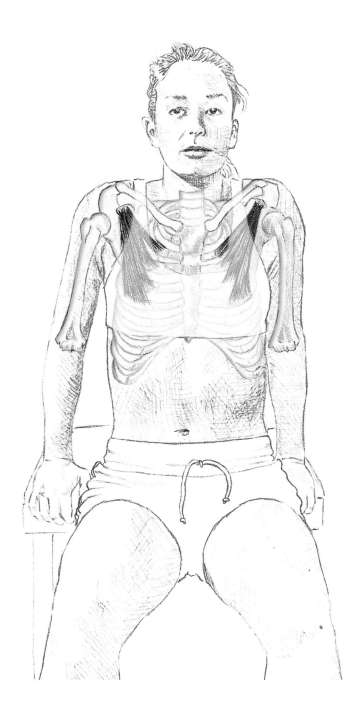

This exercise requires strong arms and a stable or attached bench. In the beginning, do this exercise very carefully. At first, you may feel the stretch in your shoulders and shoulder girdle, but this sensation should pass with time.

Precautions

Avoid this exercise if you have pain in the shoulder, neck, or wrists, or if you have difficulty holding yourself up with straight arms.

TECHNIQUE

Sit on a stable surface, such as a bench that is attached to the ground. Place your hands on the bench with your fingers pointing forward. Plant your feet on the floor before sliding your hips forward, and support yourself with your arms. Keep your upper body upright and your abs tight to maintain balance.

Stretch for 5 to 10 seconds by relaxing the shoulder muscles so that the shoulders and the shoulder girdle move up. Stop when you feel a slight stretch in the muscle on the front of the chest. Relax the muscle for 5 to 10 seconds.

Resist by using your shoulder girdle to lift your upper body about 2 inches (5 cm). Relax the muscles for 5 to 10 seconds.

Deepen the stretch by slowly letting your upper body sink down again until you reach a new ending point.

Repeat two or three times.

Common Mistakes
• Keeping the arms slightly bent
• Failing to relax the shoulder fully

Comments

Since other muscles can inhibit the movement, the lower part of your trapezius can be too tight, causing pain in the inside joint of the clavicle. Try stretching the pectoralis major before doing the exercise.

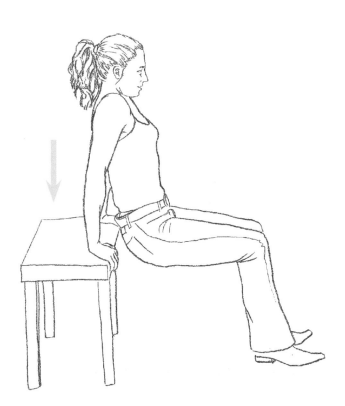

Make sure that the support surface is solid and that your arms are perfectly straight. Allow your body to slowly sink so that the shoulder rises.

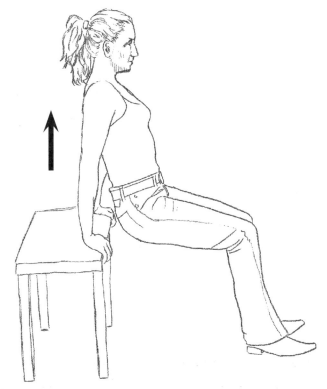

Resist by pressing your upper body about 2 inches (5 cm) toward the ceiling.

MIDDLE TRAPEZIUS AND RHOMBOIDS
(STANDING VERSION)

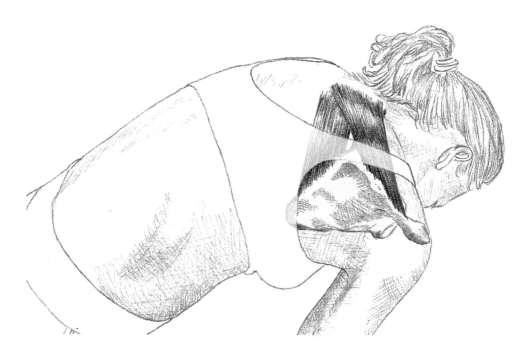

The force in this exercise is necessary because the muscles between the shoulder blades can be really tight. However, there is one problem. To do this exercise correctly, you must be able to really tighten up your abs so that you do not injure your lower back. If you feel a twinge in your lower back, you might want to try the next exercise instead. The purpose of this exercise is to use the arm to pull the shoulder blade as far forward and to the side as possible.

MUSCLE FACTS

The middle section of the trapezius is on the surface of the muscular system. It runs from processes on the spine to a point on the far end of the shoulder blade. The rhomboids, major and minor, are situated below the trapezius. They run from the processes on the spine to the inner edge of the shoulder blade. These muscles forcefully bring the shoulder blades together and stabilize the shoulder girdle.

Causes of Tightness

Bad posture makes these muscles work statically to protect the ligaments of the spine and the discs.

A shortened chest muscle can place a demand on these muscles that surpasses their capability.

Symptoms of Tightness
• Pain and aching between the shoulder blades
• Aching toward the front of the shoulder
• Numbness between the shoulder blades

Precautions

Avoid this exercise if you have pain in the lower back or in the shoulder joint.

TECHNIQUE

Stand with your right foot on a steady bench or chair and your left foot on the floor. Your left leg should be slightly bent. Cross your right arm over your legs and grab the left side of the chair. Place your hand about 4 inches (10 cm) in front of your left knee, positioning your knuckles to the left. Rest your left hand on your left thigh, just above the knee. Keeping your abs tight, let your head hang down.

Without letting go of the chair, slowly and carefully stand up by extending your right hip joint and your left knee joint. Stretch the muscles in this manner for 5 to 10 seconds. You can increase the stretch by pushing your left hand down your thigh. Continue until you feel a stretch or slight sting between the shoulder blades and the spine on your right side. Relax the muscles for 5 to 10 seconds.

Resist by carefully using your arm to pull yourself toward the chair. Keeping your upper body stationary, stretch the muscles for 5 to 10 seconds. Next, relax the muscles for 5 to 10 seconds.

Deepen the stretch by using your hand on your thigh to push yourself up toward standing position until you reach a new ending point.

Repeat two or three times.

Common Mistakes
• Failing to relax the shoulder blades
• Keeping the hand too far forward on the bench
• Turning the body along with the movement (the back should be horizontal)

Comments
Sometimes these muscles can be so tight and shortened that it is impossible to achieve a stretch. In this case, deep-tissue massage usually helps.

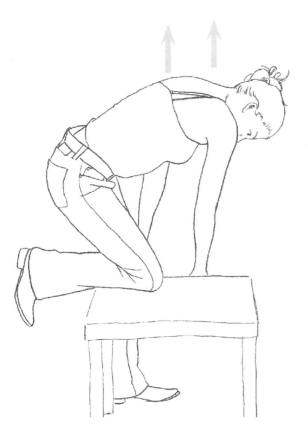

Keep your right hand about 4 inches (10 cm) in front of your right knee. Push off with your left hand and right knee. Don't forget to keep your abs tight.

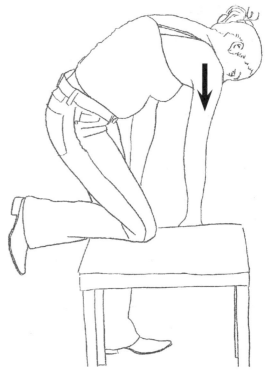

Resist by pulling yourself down toward the bench without actually moving your body.

MIDDLE TRAPEZIUS AND RHOMBOIDS
(SEATED VERSION)

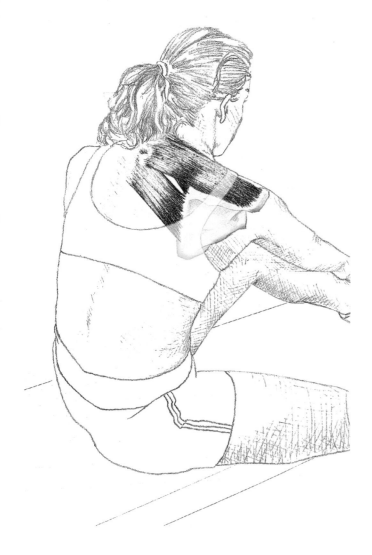

This exercise can be performed on a bench or on the floor. It can be tough if you are somewhat inflexible. If this is the case, try the previous version. As in the previous exercise, you must be able to tighten up the abs in order to protect your lower back.

Precautions

Avoid this exercise if you feel pain in the lower back or in the shoulder joint.

TECHNIQUE

Sit on a bench with your right foot on the floor and your left foot on the bench. Bend your left knee until you can reach and grab the outside of your left foot with your right hand. Place your left hand on your left thigh above the knee. Stretch by leaning your upper body backward while pushing your left hand against your thigh. Stop when you feel a slight sting between the shoulder blades and the spine on your right side. Relax the muscles for 5 to 10 seconds.

Resist for 5 to 10 seconds by using your right hand to carefully pull your upper body closer to your foot. Make sure that your upper body does not actually move. (To stretch the right side, try to turn your body to the right.) Relax the muscles for 5 to 10 seconds.

Deepen the stretch by leaning your upper body back and pushing off with your left hand until you reach a new ending point.

Repeat two or three times.

Common Mistakes

• Failing to straighten the back

• Turning the body along with the movement

Comments

These muscles can be so tight and short that you cannot achieve a stretch. Deep-tissue massage often helps. If you feel pain in your lower back, you may not be tightening your abs enough.

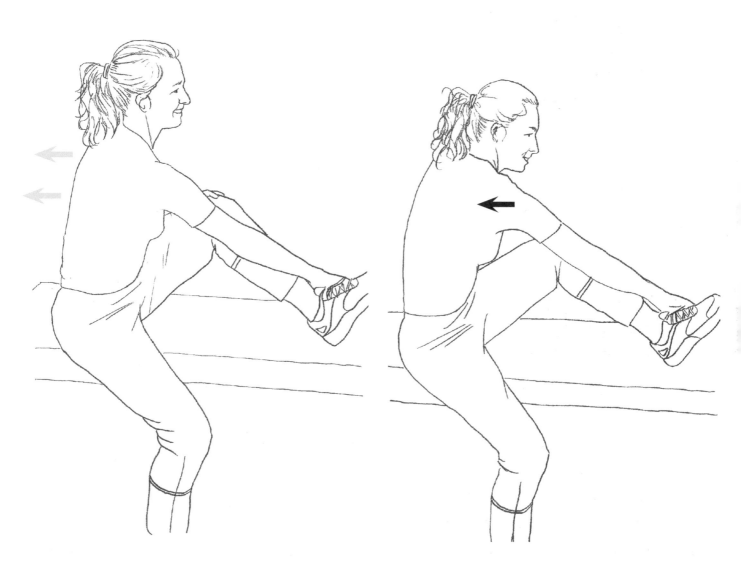

Sit up as straight as you can in the starting position. Lean your upper body backward while pushing your thigh with your left hand. Don't forget to tighten your abs.

Resist by pulling your arm and shoulder backward without actually moving your upper arm.

LATISSIMUS DORSI (STANDING VERSION)

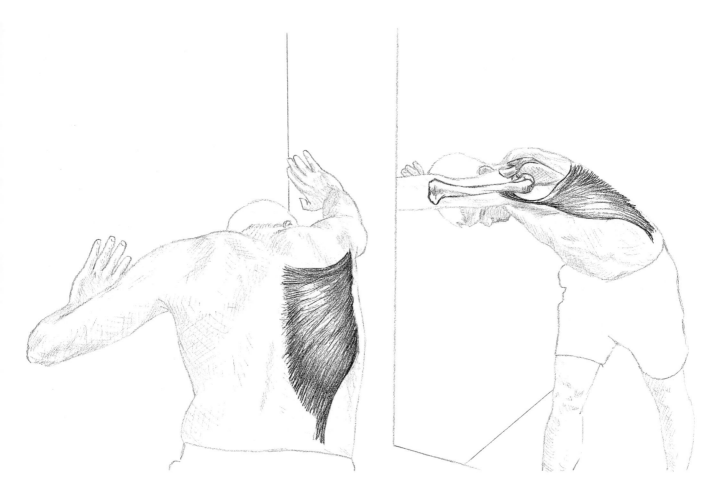

This exercise can be perceived as being technically complicated. However, once you have figured it out, you will really be able to make it work for you. It will pull and stretch the entire side of your back, all the way up to your armpit. The exercise will be easier to do if you ima-gine extending your arm and shoulder girdle as far as possible while you actively bend your body into the shape of an archer's bow.

MUSCLE FACTS

The latissimus dorsi is a wide muscle that is located very close to the skin. It starts at the iliac crest (hip) and the spine and runs around the front to the inner part of the upper arm.

The latissimus dorsi brings the arm backward and in toward the body, lowers the shoulder girdle, brings the shoulder blades together, bends the spine back-ward and sideways, and increases the arch of the back when the arms are lifted over the head.

Causes of Tightness

Since most major movements are performed with the arms below the head, this muscle commonly becomes tight and shortened from lack of exercise. It rarely becomes so tight that movement in the shoulder joint is restricted when the arms are below the level of the shoulders. However, tension in this muscle can limit movement done with the arms above the shoulder, such as cross-country skiing, gymnastics, climbing, and golf.

Symptoms of Tightness

- Difficulty working with the hands high above the head
- Pain in the shoulder joint
- Pain or ache in the lower back

Flexibility Test

Stand with your back against a wall or lie on the floor with your arms by your sides. Bring your arms up and try to reach the wall or the floor with the back of your hands. Keep your arms straight and your lower back in contact with the wall or floor at all times.

Precautions

Avoid this exercise if you have pain in the shoulder joint or in the lower back during the stretch.

TECHNIQUE

Find a door handle or something similar that is solid. It must be situated at the same height as your navel. Stand in front of the handle about arm's length away. Grab it with your right hand and take a step to the side so that your left shoulder is closer to the wall than your right one is. Bend your upper body forward so that your arm and body are lined up with each other.

Your body is now in a v-shaped angle, as seen from the side. You will have to hold the handle firmly to avoid falling backward.

Reach your right leg backward and slightly to the left. From behind, your leg, body, and arm should look like an archer's bow. Place your left hand on the door or wall, slightly to the left of your right hand. Your left arm should be slightly bent so you can use it to push off.

Stretch for 5 to 10 seconds by pushing yourself away from the wall with your left hand, increasing the bend of the bow, until you find a slight sting in the side of your back. Relax the muscle for 5 to 10 seconds.

Resist for 5 to 10 seconds by bringing your right arm to the side. Do not let go of the handle or allow your body to move. Relax your body for 5 to 10 seconds.

Deepen the stretch by increasing the bend of the bow, continuing to push off from the door or wall, until you reach a new ending point.

Repeat two or three times.

Common Mistakes

- Standing too far away from the door or handle
- Failing to bend the arm that is pushing off enough to get adequate push
- Failing to keep the shoulder joint open (straight)

Comments

If you are struggling with this exercise, ask somebody to check your starting position. To increase the stretch, grab the handle from the bottom instead. If you have trouble pushing off, stand closer to the wall.

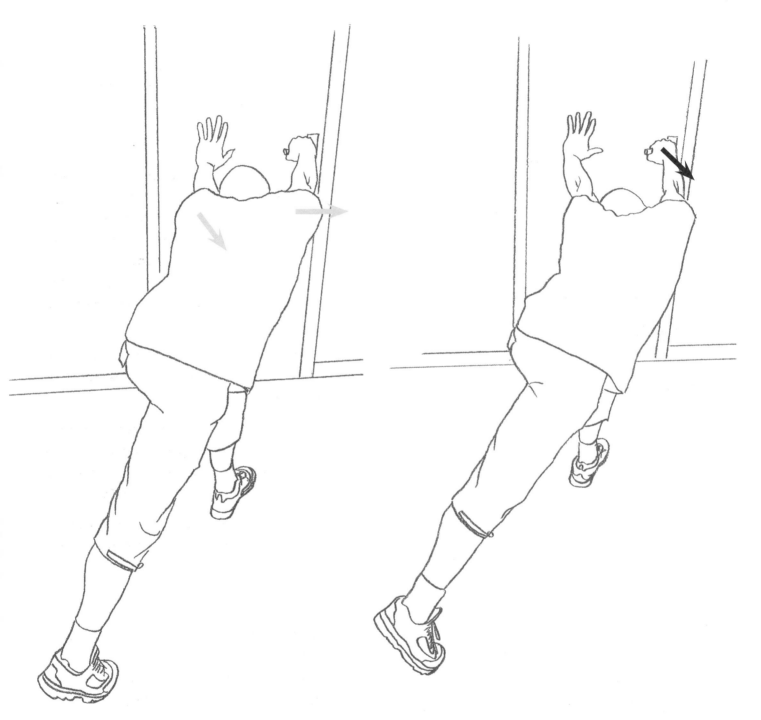

Make sure your left foot is far enough forward that you can push yourself backward. Push off with your left leg and your left hand.

Resist by bringing your right hand to the right without actually moving your body.

LATISSIMUS DORSI (SEATED VERSION)

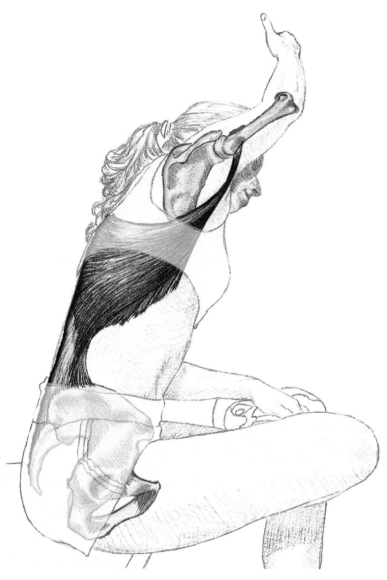

Precautions

Avoid this exercise if you have pain in the knee or in the back during the stretch.

TECHNIQUE

Sit on the chair with your right side facing the desk. Plant your feet wide apart on the floor. Put your right leg over your left leg so that your ankle rests on your thigh, and then place your right knee under the desk. Sit with your back perfectly straight and your abs tight. Lift your right arm above your head so that your upper arm touches your ear. It should rest against your head and cheek.

Stretch for 5 to 10 seconds by bending your upper body straight to the left. Try to reach up and to the left for 5 to 10 seconds.

Resist by either pushing your right knee against the desk or trying to pull your upper body up toward a straight position for 5 to 10 seconds. You can combine both if you like. Relax the muscle for 5 to 10 seconds.

Deepen the stretch by allowing gravity to pull the body to the side until you reach a new ending point.

Repeat two or three times.

Common Mistakes

- Tightening other muscles too much to allow you to sit upright
- Leaning forward instead of to the side
- Failing to bring the arm up high enough

Comments

This is a technically difficult exercise that will require some practice before it feels right. Fix your feet solidly on the floor so that you can guide the exercise with support. Sometimes it helps to stretch the quadratus lumborum first.

This exercise is well suited for somebody who is fairly flexible. It is also perfect for doing at work. To perform this exercise, you must be able to sit totally upright in the starting position. Before you are used to this exercise, take it slowly and carefully, using one of your hands for support. If not, you risk using too much force in the stretch.

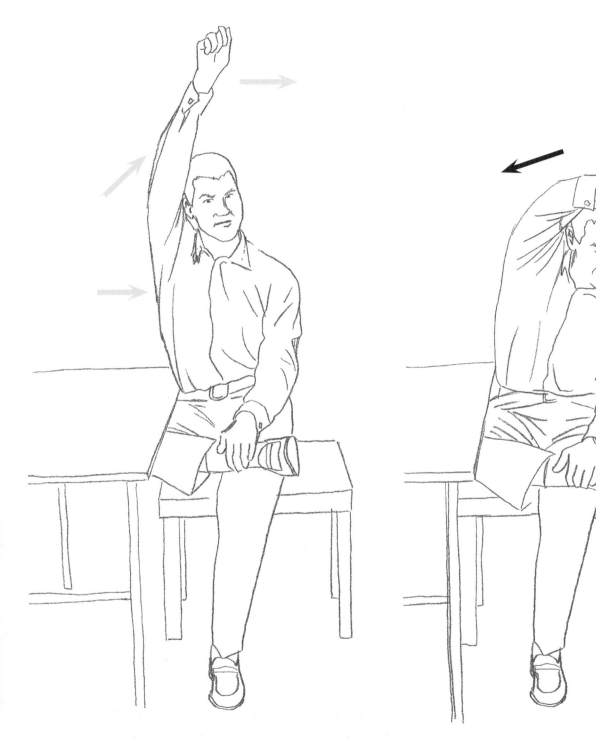

Position your leg under the table top and raise your arm as high as you can. Leaning your upper body to the left, reach your arm forward and to the side.

Resist by carefully pushing your knee against the table top or by raising your upper body a couple of inches (5 cm).

INFRASPINATUS (VERSION 1)

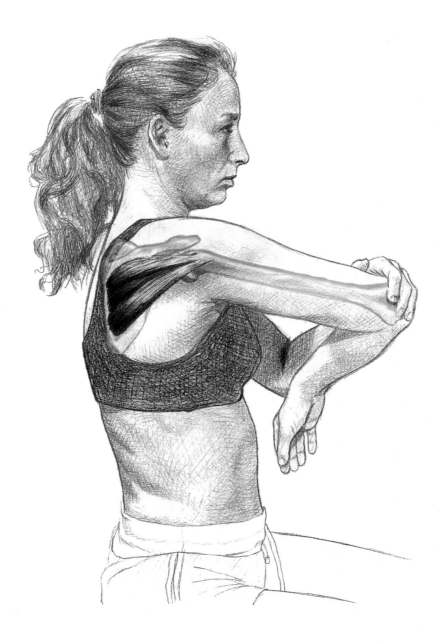

The infraspinatus is one of the most important muscles for avoiding or minimizing pain in the shoulder area. Since it is known to be a sensitive muscle, proceed with caution. Even if you do not feel a real stretch in the muscle, the exercise can still be of value. The muscle rotates the upper arm internally, which stretches the shoulder externally. To get the desired effect from this exercise, you should not raise or lower your elbow during the stretch. It is also important that you not move too vigorously when creating resistance.

MUSCLE FACTS

The infraspinatus is located close to the skin and runs from the shoulder blade to the outside of the upper arm. Its main function is to rotate the arm externally in the shoulder joint. It also stabilizes the shoulder by coordinating and making small adjustments to the joint's movements.

Causes of Tightness

The infraspinatus works statically whenever the arm is moved. It can become very tight and shortened from working on a keyboard. It can be overused during strength training, especially by pushing exercises like the bench press. It can also be strained by exercises that involve pushing and pulling behind the neck.

Symptoms of Tightness

- Experiencing pain either locally or across the shoulder blade
- Stabbing pain in the front of the shoulder
- Pain that radiates down the arm, forearm, and hand

Flexibility Test

Lie on the floor on your front or stand with your front against a wall. Reach behind you and place a finger in a belt loop or in the waistline of your pants as far back as possible. If you are lying down, gravity should pull your elbow down to touch the floor. If you are standing, you should be able to pull your elbow forward to touch the wall.

Precautions

Avoid this exercise if you feel pain in the front of your shoulder during the stretch. If you have pain after the stretch, be a little more careful next time.

TECHNIQUE

This exercise can be done while either sitting or standing. Hold your right arm straight out in front of you, and then bring your forearm toward your chest to create a 90-degree angle in your elbow. Grab your right elbow with your left hand so that your left forearm rests on top of your right forearm. Relax your right arm, holding the position with your left arm. Relax and lower your shoulder.

Stretch the muscle for 5 to 10 seconds by pushing your right hand down with your left forearm, keeping your right elbow in place. Relax the muscle for 5 to 10 seconds.

Create resistance by carefully pushing your right hand up against your left forearm. Relax the muscle for 5 to 10 seconds.

Deepen the stretch by pushing your hand and forearm down until you reach a new ending point.

Repeat two or three times.

Common Mistakes

- Failing to completely relax the shoulders
- Moving too quickly
- Tightening other muscles surrounding the shoulder joint too much

Comments

It is hard to really feel a good stretch in the infraspinatus muscle. Sometimes you can only feel it in the front of the shoulder instead of across the shoulder blade. To increase your awareness of this muscle, train the muscles in the chest and back to increase the blood flow to these regions before stretching the infraspinatus. If you still having difficulty, try deep-tissue massage in the area before stretching. You can also try to open up the shoulder joint before starting the rotation by pulling your elbow forward with your left hand.

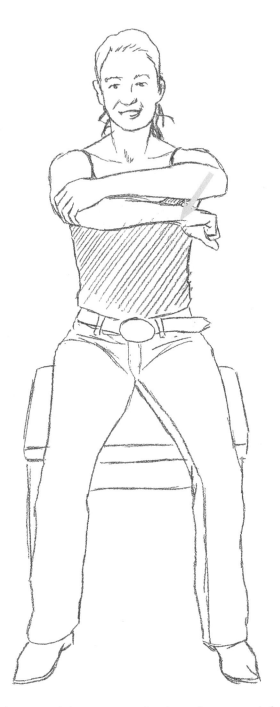

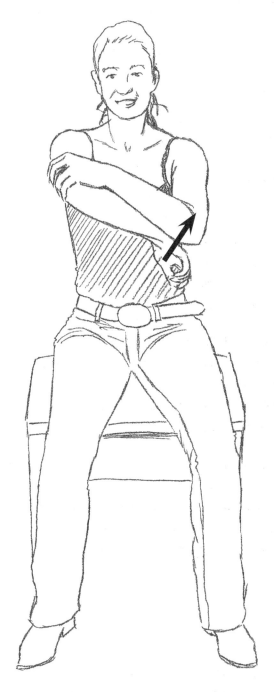

Relax your right arm completely and use your left arm to lift it up. Rotate the arm internally with your left elbow.

Resist by pressing your right hand against your left elbow.

INFRASPINATUS (VERSION 2)

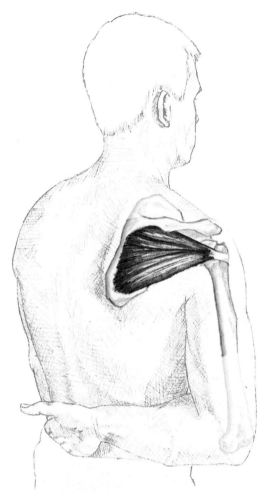

This exercise, which is usually referred to as the police hold, is a very forceful stretch for the infraspinatus. Proceed carefully, taking into account the size of this muscle in relation to your body weight. Make sure that you are well balanced and that you do not add more force than what is provided by gravity while leaning your body. When you have reached the starting position, the goal of this exercise is to move your elbow forward while shifting your body backward. The resistance (in this case, the door frame) should rest against the back of your elbow.

Precautions

Avoid this exercise if you have pain in the shoulder during or immediately after the exercise.

TECHNIQUE

Stand in a doorway with one leg in front of the other. Put your hand behind your back and place one finger in the belt loop or waistline of your pants. Lean the back of your elbow against the door frame. Stretch the muscle for 5 to 10 seconds by carefully leaning your upper body backward until you feel a slight stretch or sting in the muscle. If you are doing this correctly, your elbow should come forward. Relax the muscle for 5 to 10 seconds.

Deepen the stretch by leaning your body backward and bringing your elbow forward until you reach a new ending point.

Repeat two or three times.

Common Mistakes
- Failing to fully relax the shoulder
- Tensing the muscles around the shoulder joint
- Touching the door frame with too much of your arm

Comments

If you have pain or difficulty reaching the muscle, try holding a belt loop that is closer to the side. Make sure that your elbow alone touches the door frame rather than your entire arm.

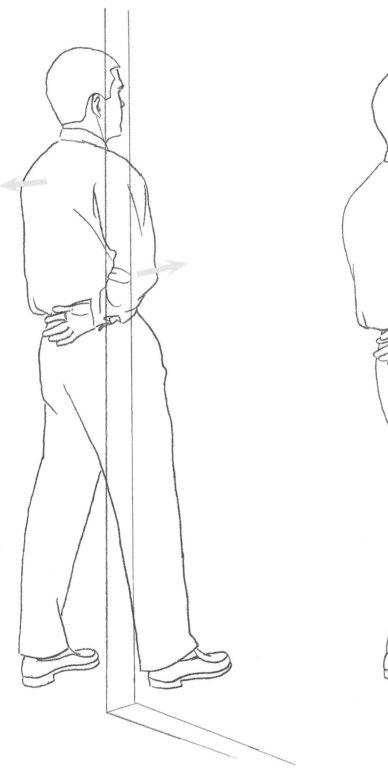

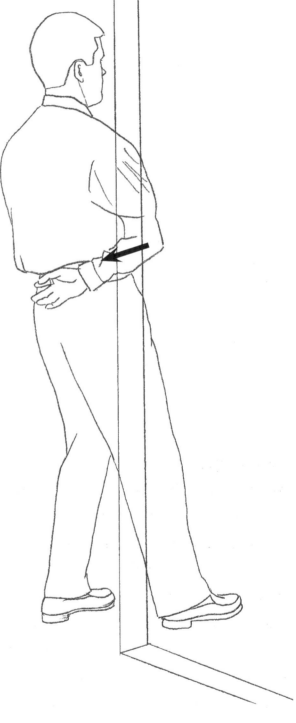

Place your elbow in front of a door frame. Slowly lean your upper body backward so that your elbow is brought forward.

Resist by carefully pressing your elbow back against the door frame.

TERES MAJOR

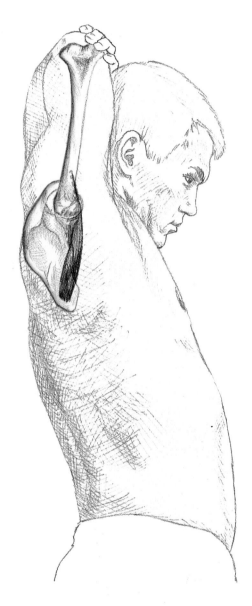

Since the teres major has the same functions in the shoulder joint that the latissimus dorsi does, it is therefore stretched by the same exercises, as seen on pages 52 and 55. This exercise is a little more specific to the teres major because it anchors the shoulder blade against the wall.

MUSCLE FACTS

The teres major runs from the lower, triangular part of the shoulder blade to its points of insertion on the inside of the upper arm, next to the latissimus dorsi. It moves the arm toward the body from all positions in front of or to the side of the body. It also helps rotate the upper arm inward.

Causes of Tightness

Static work for long periods can make this muscle tighten up, but this tension rarely impedes movements performed below the shoulders. However, tension can really impede movements done above the head. Examples include movements in cross-country skiing, gymnastics, climbing, and golf.

Symptoms of Tightness

• Pain radiating down the arm
• Numbness in the arm and fingers
• Loss of strength when moving the arms above the head

Precautions

Avoid this exercise if you have pain in the shoulder or the neck.

TECHNIQUE

Stand with your right side facing the wall and your feet a little more than one foot (30 cm) away from the wall. Bring your right arm above your head and bend your elbow to a 90-degree angle. Carefully lean your right side against the wall so that only your shoulder blade touches the wall. Grab your right elbow with your left hand.

Stretch for 5 to 10 seconds by pulling your elbow behind your head to the left until you feel resistance or a slight sting just below the outside of your shoulder. Relax the muscle for 5 to 10 seconds.

Resist by carefully bringing your elbow toward the wall while resisting with your left hand. Relax the muscle for 5 to 10 seconds.

Deepen the stretch by pulling your elbow behind your head until you reach a new ending point.

Repeat two or three times.

Common Mistakes

- Standing too close to the wall to anchor the shoulder blade
- Failing to bring your arm behind your head due to stiffness in the shoulder joint or related muscles

Comments

If you find this exercise difficult, try stretching the latissimus dorsi and the pectoralis major first.

Bring your right arm behind your head. Use your other hand to pull your elbow to the left. Resist by pressing your right elbow into your left hand.

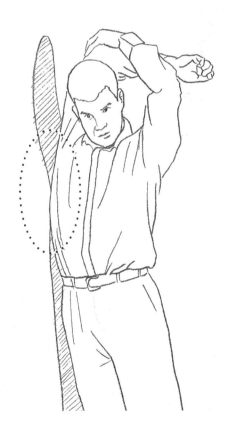

It is important to anchor your shoulder blade against the wall.

SUPRASPINATUS (VERSION 1)

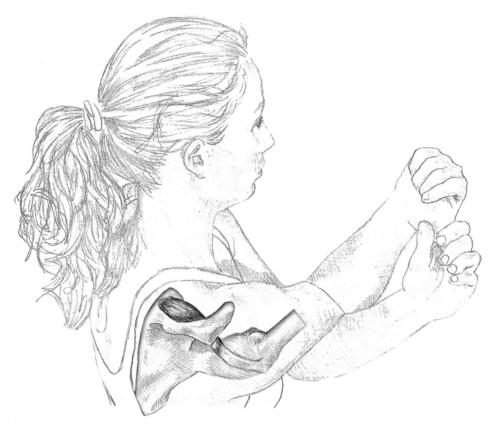

This is one of the most difficult exercises, both because it can be difficult to feel the stretch in this muscle and because your arms might be too large. If this is the case, try the next exercise instead. Once again, you must realize that you are dealing with a small muscle. Forcefully pulling is not a good idea. Make small adjustments to the starting position and carefully feel your way through the movement. Do not give up just because you cannot get the hang of it right away.

MUSCLE FACTS

The supraspinatus is a relatively small muscle that is located below the middle part of the trapezius. It runs from the top of the shoulder blade, below the protrusions on the outside of the shoulder blade, and attaches to the outside of the upper arm. The supraspinatus has a very important function: It makes sure that the upper arm is pulled in toward the shoulder blade during shoulder movements in the shoulder joint. Without this action, the other muscles around the shoulder would not be able to do their work. It also aids in rotating the arm externally and lifting the arm out to the side.

Causes of Tightness

The supraspinatus is always at work when the upper arm is in motion. Therefore, it is rarely at rest. It can also get pinched or injured by repeated movements above the shoulder. Cleaning windows or painting ceilings or walls can cause trouble for this muscle.

Symptoms of Tightness

• Local pain over the muscle and on the outside of the shoulder

• Local pain when raising the elbow above the shoulders

The muscle is also considered to be partially involved when pain in the shoulder and neck radiates down into the arms and hands. It is also involved in cases of tennis elbow. In this case, the pain is located on the outside of the elbow.

Precautions
Avoid this exercise if you have pain in the shoulder or the wrist.

TECHNIQUE
This exercise can be done either while sitting or standing. Put your right arm in front of your body (as if arm wrestling), maintaining a 90-degree angle in the elbow. Next, bring your elbow toward the midline of your body to a position in front of your solar plexus. Place your left arm under the right so that your right elbow rests on the front of your left elbow. Grab your right thumb with your left hand. Your arms should now be crossed, with your right forearm pointing straight up. Relax your shoulder and arm.

Carefully stretch the muscle by pulling your right thumb with your left hand so that your arm rotates externally.

Slightly extend your elbow as you rotate your arm. Stop when you feel a slight stretch or sting in your right shoulder. Relax the muscle for 5 to 10 seconds.

Resist by trying to rotate your arm internally (as in arm wrestling) without actually moving your arm until the stinging in the muscle diminishes. Relax the muscle for 5 to 10 seconds.

Deepen the stretch by continuing to rotate the arm externally until you reach a new ending point.

Repeat two or three times.

Common Mistakes
- Bending the elbow too much
- Failing to position the elbow in front of the solar plexus
- Failing to relax the shoulder and arm

Comments
Although it can be hard to feel any action in this muscle, you may still be achieving a stretch. If you find this exercise difficult due to inflexibility or too much muscle mass, you might want to try the following exercise.

Make sure that your elbow stays directly in front of your body throughout the exercise. Carefully stretch by pulling your thumb.

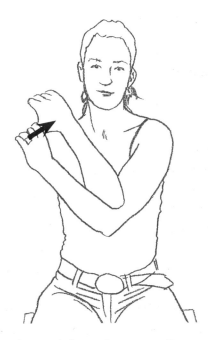

Resist with your left arm by pretending you are arm wrestling with your right arm.

SUPRASPINATUS (VERSION 2)

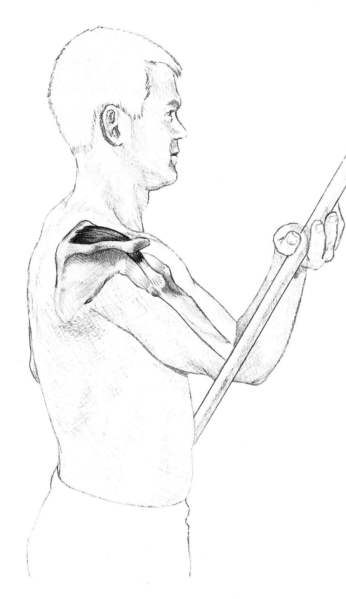

TECHNIQUE

Put your right arm in front of your body (as if arm wrestling), forming a 90-degree angle in your elbow. Next, bring your elbow toward the midline of your body to a position in front of your solar plexus. Turn the back of your hand toward the front and grab a small stick with your thumb and index finger. Allow the stick to hang down along the outside of your right arm.

Place your left arm under the right, grab the stick, and pull it up toward your left hip until you feel the stretch through your shoulder. Relax your shoulder and arm for 5 to 10 seconds.

Resist by trying to rotate your arm internally (as in arm wrestling) without actually moving it until the stinging in the muscle diminishes. Relax the muscle for 5 to 10 seconds.

Deepen the stretch by pulling the stick until you reach a new ending point.

Repeat two or three times.

Common Mistakes
- Failing to relax the shoulder and arm
- Failing to position the elbow in front of the solar plexus
- Lack of flexibility in the muscles surrounding the shoulder joint

This is a great alternative for people who struggle with the previous exercise due to inflexibility or injury. The exercise is essentially the same, but you use a small stick as a prop. Remember that leverage increases the force, so be aware of how you feel and proceed with caution.

Precautions
Avoid this exercise if you have pain in the wrist or in the shoulder.

Comments
If you don't have access to a stick, use a towel instead.

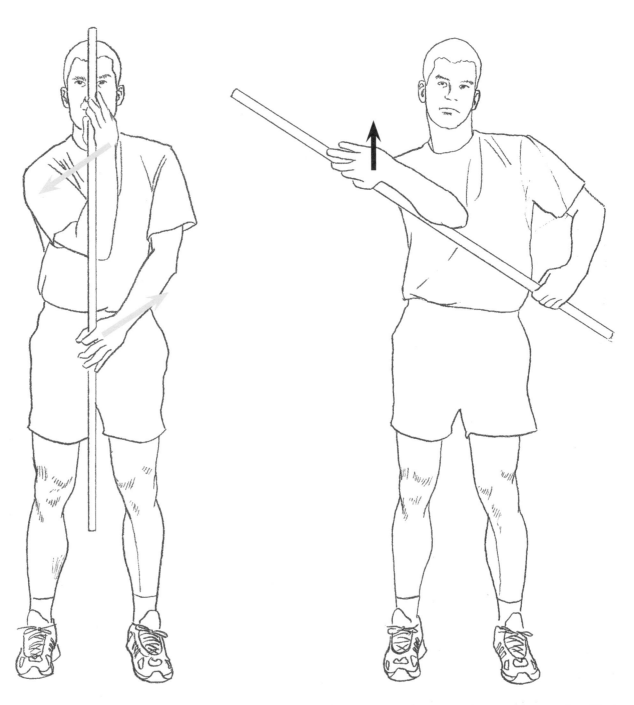

Keep your elbow right in the middle of your body, just above your navel. Carefully pull the stick back and to the side.

Create resistance by pretending to arm wrestle with your right arm while using your left hand to keep the stick from moving.

GLUTEUS MAXIMUS

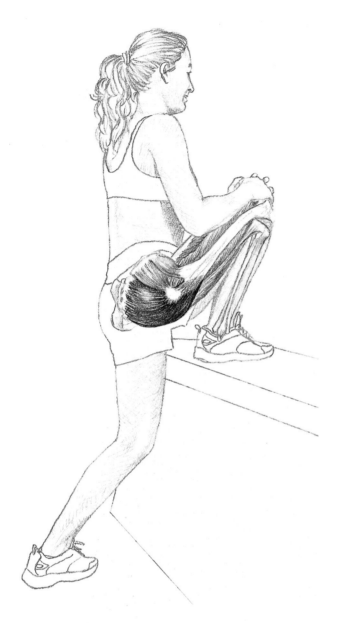

MUSCLE FACTS

The gluteus maximus is one of the largest muscles in the body. It is located below the surface muscles, running from the coccyx and the iliac crest and attaching to the outside of the top of the femur. The gluteus maximus extends the hip joint, rotates the leg externally, and decreases the arch in the small of your back.

Causes of Tightness

The upper part of the gluteus maximus becomes tight more easily than the lower part does. Sitting for extended periods with your legs externally rotated, such as while driving, can cause muscle tension. The gluteus maximus is also activated during squatting motions. Athletes in sports like running, skating, and skiing are often affected.

Symptoms of Tightness

- Ache or pain in the small of the back or either on the back side or outside of the leg
- Difficulty bending forward

Flexibility Test

Lie on your back, bend your knee, and move it up toward your chest. You should reach an angle about 120 degrees from the floor.

Precautions

Avoid this exercise if you have pain in the knee.

People with a normal range of motion are not likely to feel any stretch in this muscle. However, if you are somewhat inflexible, this can be a good exercise to do before stretching the other muscles in your buttocks, such as the piriformis and the gluteus medius.

TECHNIQUE

Stand in front of a sturdy chair or stool. The more flexible you are, the higher the chair or stool should be. Put your right foot on the chair or stool. Try to keep your back as straight as possible and your abs tight.

Stretch the muscle for 5 to 10 seconds by bending your left leg until you feel the stretch over your right buttock. Relax the muscle for 5 to 10 seconds.

Resist by pushing your front leg down for 5 to 10 seconds.

Deepen the stretch by continuing to bend your left leg until you reach a new ending point.

Repeat two or three times.

Common Mistakes
• Placing the front foot too low
• Failing to keep the back upright
• Turning the knee out during the stretch

Comments
Sometimes it is difficult to feel a stretch in this muscle if it is already flexible. If so, try stretching the piriformis or the gluteus medius instead.

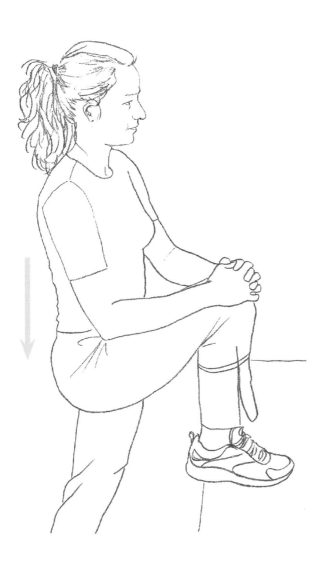

Adjust the height of the surface depending on your level of flexibility. Keep your back straight as you bend your left knee with control.

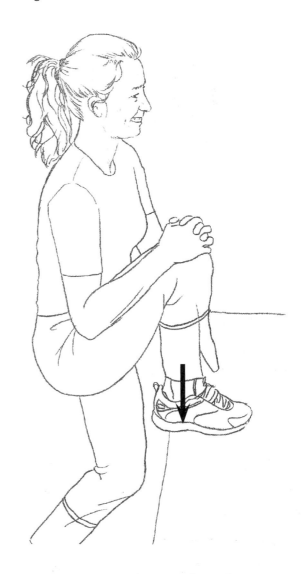

Resist by pressing your foot into the surface.

GLUTEUS MEDIUS AND MINIMUS

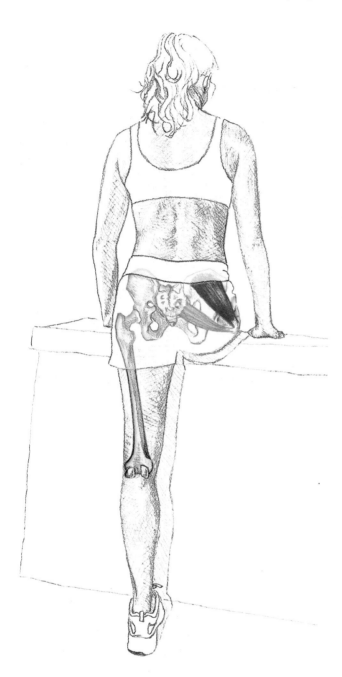

These muscles work constantly during walking or running, which means they need to be stretched often. Since they rotate the hip backward, decreasing the arch of the back, you should try to increase the arch throughout this exercise to achieve a stretch. These muscles can negatively affect the small of your back if you do keep your abs tight.

MUSCLE FACTS

The gluteus medius and minimus are layered, with the gluteus medius entirely covering the gluteus minimus. They are situated on the outside of the hip bone and run down to the bump on the outer top of the femur. The main job of the gluteus medius and minimus is to keep the pelvis straight, especially while walking, running, and standing on one leg. They also help move the leg out to the side and rotate it both internally and externally.

Causes of Tightness

Most people favor a certain side of the body, leaning or tilting the hip toward it. This habit creates static tension on the favored side. Sometimes a difference in leg length causes one hip to hang out. Weight is usually borne on the shorter leg. Injuries might also prompt people to bear more weight with one leg than the other.

Symptoms of Tightness

• Local pain in the muscles and in the small of the back
• Aches radiating down the leg (false sciatica)

Precautions

Avoid this exercise if you have pain on the inside or the outside of the knee.

TECHNIQUE

Look for a table, desk, or another flat surface at the same height as your groin.

Put your right foot on the table so that your right knee is positioned in front of your navel and your foot is to the left of your left hip.

Turn your pelvis to face straight forward. Imagine that your leg creates a triangle, with your pelvis forming the base. Tighten up your abs and try to increase the arch of the lower back. Remember to keep your supporting leg perfectly straight.

Stretch for 5 to 10 seconds by slowly leaning your upper body forward while maintaining the arch. Stop when you feel a stretch or a slight sting across your right buttock. Relax the muscles for 5 to 10 seconds.

Resist by pushing your knee down toward the surface for 5 to 10 seconds. Relax the muscles for 5 to 10 seconds.

Deepen the stretch by leaning your upper body forward while maintaining the arch until you reach a new ending point.

Repeat two or three times.

Common Mistakes

- Failing to maintain the arch
- Allowing the knee to slide out of the position in front of the navel

Comments

If you have difficulty keeping your body up, support yourself on the table with your fingertips.

If you feel pain in the groin on the side you are stretching, slightly move your knee out to the side. If you have trouble maintaining the arch, the muscle may be too tight or the surface may be too high.

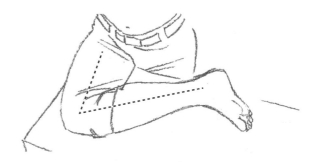

Your knee should be positioned directly in front of your navel.

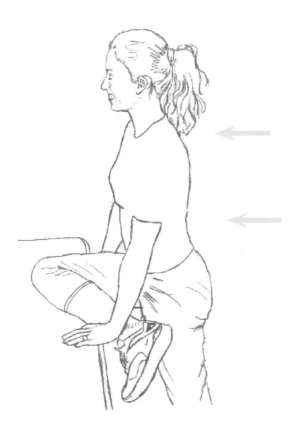

The surface should be at the height of your groin. Make sure that your hips are parallel with the surface. Don't forget to keep your abs tight and your back completely straight as you lean your upper body forward.

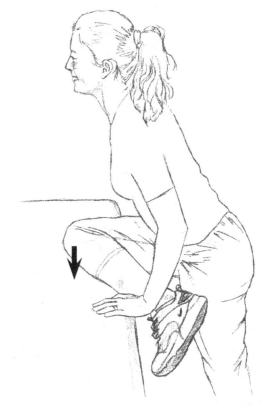

Resist by pressing your right knee into the surface.

PIRIFORMIS (STANDING VERSION)

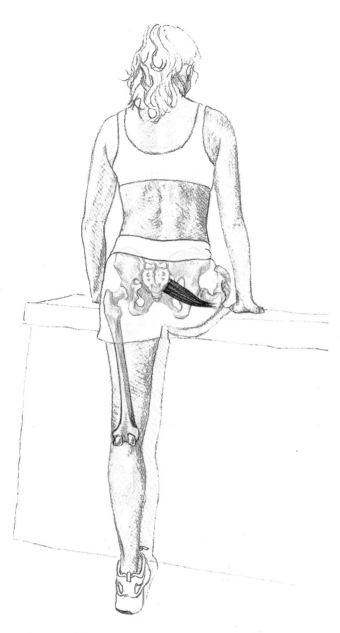

MUSCLE FACTS

The piriformis, which is situated under the gluteus maximus, belongs to the deep muscles that affect the hip joint. It runs from the front of the sacrum to the large process on the top of the femur, or the greater trochanter. The main function of the piriformis is to rotate the leg externally when the hip joint is extended (when standing). When the hip joint is flexed more than 60 degrees, this muscle causes internal rotation instead.

Causes of Tightness

The piriformis becomes tight and shortened from too much sitting, both short term and long term. Think of all the sitting that you have done over the years! Sitting with your feet wide apart creates an external rotation in the hips that affects the muscle even more. The piriformis is also greatly affected by its antagonists, such as the hip flexors, which increase the demand on the muscle when they are tight. The hip flexors also rotate the leg externally, causing the piriformis to be shortened passively.

Flexibility Test

Test 1

Lie on your front with your knees together and bend one leg to a 90-degree angle. Let your lower leg fall to the outside, keeping the opposite hip on the floor. The angle between your lower leg and the floor should be about 45 to 50 degrees. Both legs should have the same range of movement.

Test 2

Sit on a chair with your legs together and your back straight. Put one leg on the other knee, pointing the heel of your foot at your groin, and let the knee of the elevated leg drop out to the side. Your lower leg should now be in a horizontal position.

Repeat with the other leg and compare the range of movement of each leg. Take care to sit in the same position during the test.

The piriformis is a muscle that everybody should stretch on a daily basis. This muscle causes pain in both the small of the back and in the leg. Its special position also causes it to occasionally be penetrated by the sciatic nerve. If this muscle tightens up, it can directly push on the nerve, causing local pain or radiating pain down the leg (false sciatica).

Symptoms of Tightness

- Local ache or pain in the buttocks
- Numbness and pain running down from the back of the thigh to the back of the knee
- Pain and ache in the small of the back
- Pain on the outside of the knee, also called runner's knee

Precautions

Avoid this exercise if you feel pain on the inside or the outside of the knee or if you have discomfort in the groin area during the stretch.

TECHNIQUE

Use a surface that is the same height as your groin. Depending on your height, you might be able to use the kitchen table, the kitchen island, or an ironing board propped against a door opening. Put your right leg up so that your right knee is positioned straight in front of your right hip. Make sure that the knee is bent to 90 degrees. Your thigh and pelvis should also form a right angle.

From above, your pelvis and leg should resemble an open square. Make sure that your supporting leg is straight and vertical.

Now, try to arch your lower back as much as possible, keeping your abs tight.

You have now reached the correct starting position.

Stretch the muscle for 5 to 10 seconds by carefully leaning your upper body forward, maintaining the arch, until you feel a slight sting across the muscle. Relax the muscle for 5 to 10 seconds.

Resist by carefully pressing your foot and knee down for 5 to 10 seconds. The stinging feeling should disappear when you resist. If it does not, you have stretched too far. Relax the muscle for 5 to 10 seconds.

Deepen the stretch by leaning your upper body forward until you feel a slight sting in the muscle again. This is your new ending point.

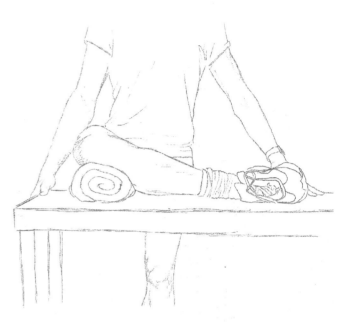

Put a towel under your knee if it does not reach the surface.

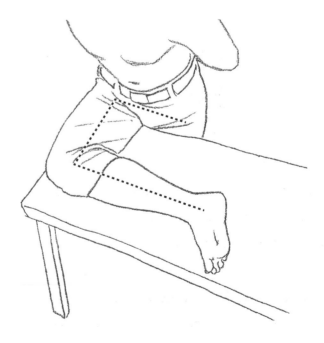

Your knee should be at a right angle, and your hips, thigh, and lower leg should form an open square.

Common Mistakes

- Moving the leg out of alignment with the groin
- Bending the knee too much
- Failing to arch the back enough
- Shifting the pelvis away from the forward position

Comments

If your groin hurts, try moving your knee to the side slightly. If your knee hurts, put a cushion under it to lend support. If you have trouble maintaining alignment, the surface is too high or too low. If this exercise is too difficult, stretch the gluteus maximus and medius for a while before coming back to this exercise. You can also try the seated version of this exercise. Feel free to grip the surface with your hands if you are struggling to keep your upper body upright.

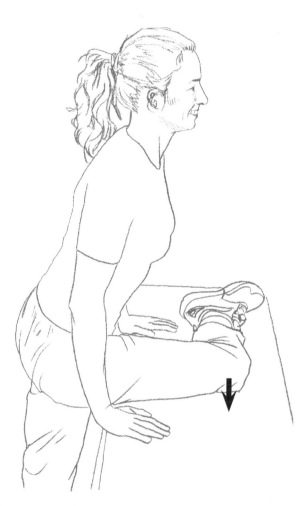

As you lean your upper body forward, maintain the arch in your lower back. Use your fingertips to support yourself. Don't forget to keep your abs tight.

Resist by pressing your right knee into the surface.

PIRIFORMIS (SEATED VERSION)

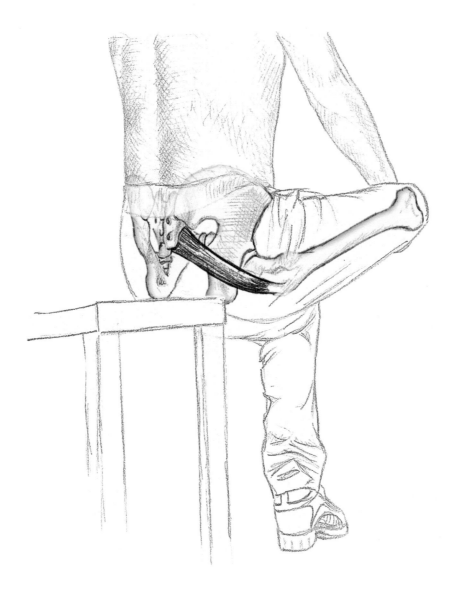

This exercise is helpful if you are having difficulty with the standing version. Maybe your muscles are too tight, making it difficult to find the correct starting position. Even if the standing version is more effective, you might also feel more comfortable doing this version.

The seated version has two options. If you are really tight, try option 2, which allows you to gradually push your knee down. If you are slightly more flexible and able to move your lower leg into a horizontal position, try option 1, which leans the upper body forward.

Precautions

Avoid this exercise if you have pain on the inside or the outside of the knee or in the small of the back during the stretch.

TECHNIQUE

The starting position for this exercise is the same as for the second flexibility test on page 72. Sit on a chair with your feet together and your back upright. Put your right leg over your left so that the outside of your right foot rests on your left thigh, just above the knee. Sit straight up, tighten your abs, and arch your lower back as much as possible. Anchor your knee by pushing down on it with one hand.

Stretch the muscle for 5 to 10 seconds by either leaning your upper body forward or pushing your knee toward the floor until you feel a slight sting in the muscle. Relax the muscle for 5 to 10 seconds.

Resist by carefully pushing your knee up against your hand for 5 to 10 seconds or by attempting to press your leg down toward your thigh for 5 to 10 seconds. Relax the muscle for 5 to 10 seconds.

Stretch by either leaning your upper body forward or by pushing the knee down with your hand until you feel the stretch in the muscle again. This is your new ending point.

Repeat two or three times.

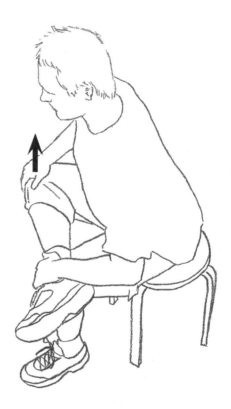

From the starting position, sit up as straight as possible and lightly press your knee down. Lean your upper body forward, maintaining the arch in your lower back.

Resist by pressing your right knee up against your hand.

Common Mistakes

- Struggling to hold the body in an upright position
- Struggling to increase and maintain the arch during the exercise
- Failing to rest the foot against the thigh, moving the pressure higher up on the lower leg
- Assuming an incorrect starting position due to inflexibility in other muscles

Comments

If you have difficulty achieving a good stretch in the muscle, try the standing version of this exercise on page 72. If you are too tight for either of these exercises, you might want to consider deep-tissue massage or ask a naprapath or physical therapist to help you with the stretch.

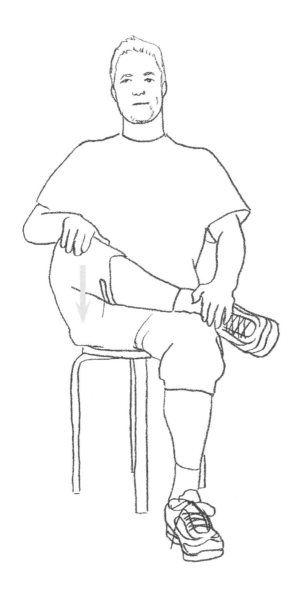

Sit with your back straight and your abs tight. Carefully press your knee down toward the floor.

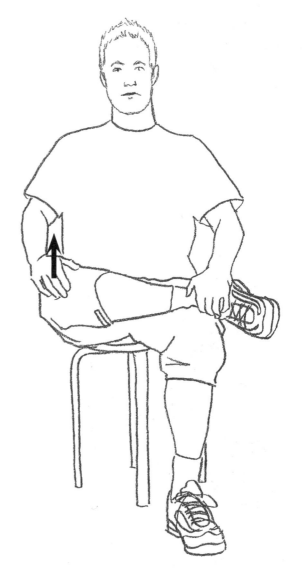

Resist by pressing your right knee against your hand.

QUADRATUS LUMBORUM (LYING VERSION)

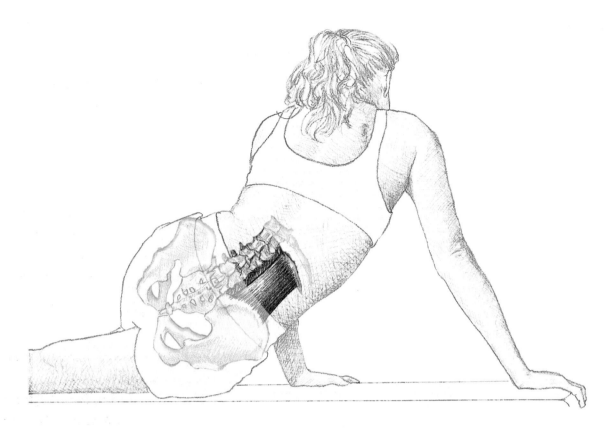

This forceful exercise demands a certain degree of strength in the arms and good body control. If you cannot maintain a perfectly straight line in your body throughout the exercise, you will not achieve a worthwhile stretch. If you have access to some kind of line or marking on the floor, use it to locate the correct starting position. Moving from the beach position to stretching can be a little tricky in the beginning, but using your left hand for assistance usually helps.

Remember that this is a forceful stretching exercise; be careful at the beginning to avoid hurting yourself.

MUSCLE FACTS

The quadratus lumborum is situated deep in your lower back, below the long, straight muscles on each side of the spine. It runs from the top edge of the hip bone and the lumbar spine and attaches to the bottom rib. The quadratus lumborum flexes the back backward and to the side, rotates the upper body, and increases the arch in the lower back.

Causes of Tightness

If you usually sleep on your side in a bed that is too soft, your quadratus lumborum can become tight and shortened on the side of your body that faces the ceiling.

Differences in leg length also cause muscle compensation in the upper body, which forces the quadratus lumborum to constantly work statically when you stand or walk.

Symptoms of Tightness

- Pain or ache in the lower back
- Pain in the lower back during forced inhalation

Precautions

Avoid this exercise if you have pain in the lower back or in the shoulder during the stretch.

TECHNIQUE

Lie on the right side of your body, supporting yourself with your forearm, in what is called the beach position. Make sure that your body is straight. Bend your left leg and pull it up as far as you can without moving your bottom leg. If your bottom leg and upper body are still in a straight line, you have reached the starting position.

Stretch for 5 to 10 seconds by placing your right hand on the floor exactly where you had placed your right elbow before. Slowly straighten your arm. Feel free to use your left hand for support until you find your balance. Stop the movement when you feel a slight sting or stretch in the right side of your waist. Relax the muscle for 5 to 10 seconds.

Resist by pressing your bottom leg into the floor for 5 to 10 seconds.

Deepen the stretch by continuing to straighten your arm or by moving it closer to your hip until you reach a new ending point.

Repeat two or three times.

Common Mistakes

- Changing the starting position so that the bottom hip is no longer in line with the rest of the body
- Failing to pull the knee up high enough
- Rolling the upper body forward and stretching the obliques instead

Comments

If you are experiencing pain in the wrist, turn your hand so that your fingers point away from you. If you are not able to push yourself up with your arm, try putting your forearm on a raised surface instead. A couple of pillows or phone books usually work well to elevate the arm.

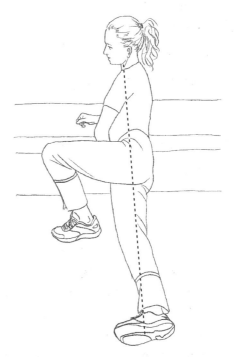

If you are not able to push up while keeping your arm straight, put your forearm on a raised surface.

Make sure that your upper body and leg are in a straight line.

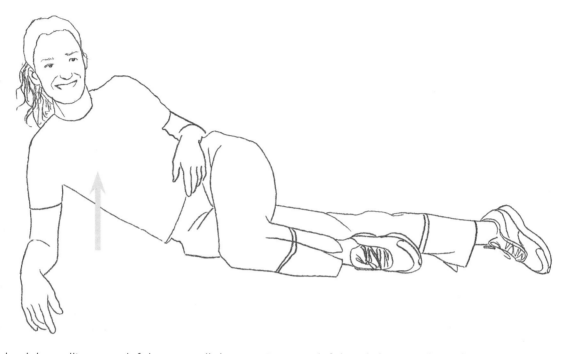

Protect your back by pulling your left knee up all the way. Put your left hand down and carefully straighten your arm.

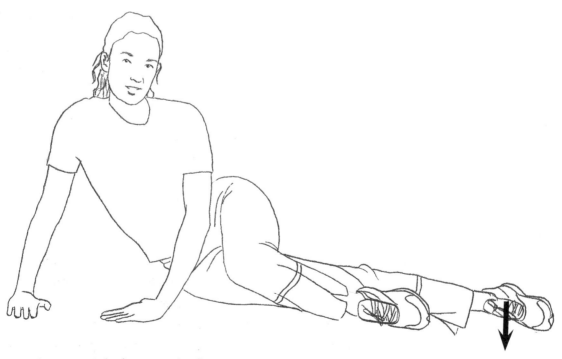

Resist by pressing your right foot into the floor.

QUADRATUS LUMBORUM (SEATED VERSION)

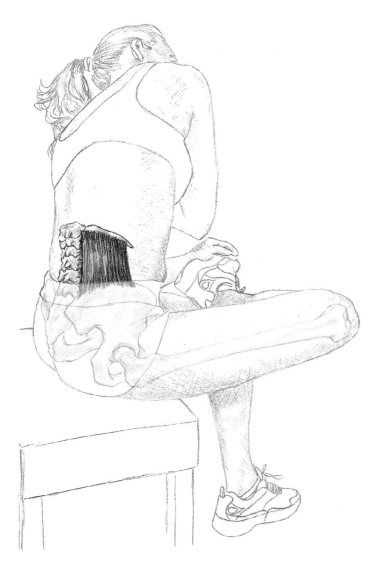

This exercise can be a good alternative to the supine version. However, it does require a certain amount of flexibility and balance. It works well when sitting at your desk at work. If you have problems with your groin muscles, you need to be especially careful. Make sure that you keep your abs tight.

Precautions

Avoid this exercise if you have problems balancing or if you have pain in the groin or knee.

TECHNIQUE

The starting position for this exercise is the same as the one in the second flexibility test for the piriformis on page 72. Sit on a chair with your feet together and your back straight. Put your right foot on your left leg, resting the outside of your right ankle on your left thigh just above your knee. Position your right knee under a tabletop so that it is anchored and cannot move upward. Next, put your right hand on your left shoulder.

Stretch for 5 to 10 seconds by carefully leaning your upper body to the left. Continue until you feel a slight sting in the muscle. Relax the muscle for 5 to 10 seconds.

Resist by carefully pushing your right knee against the tabletop for 5 to 10 seconds. You can also try to carefully raise your upper body about a 1/2 inch (1 cm) at this time. Relax the muscle for 5 to 10 seconds.

Deepen the stretch by continuing to lean your upper body to the side until you reach a new ending point.

Repeat two or three times.

Common Mistakes
- Leaning the body too far forward
- Tightening the gluteal muscles too much, making it difficult to sit upright

Comments

If you have a hard time attaining a stretch, try rotating your upper body slightly to the right while stretching the right side. If your knee hurts, try putting something soft between your knee and the tabletop. If you are a little unsure of your balance, place a chair next to you so you have something to lean on.

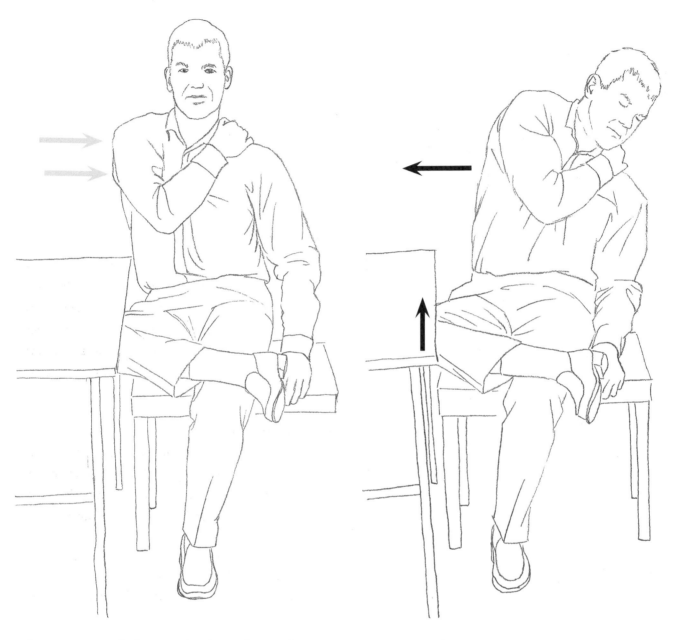

Position your right knee under the surface and raise your upper body as far as you can. Slightly rotate your upper body to the left and then lean to the side.

Resist by carefully pressing your knee against the surface or by lifting your upper body a couple of inches (5 cm).

PSOAS AND ILIACUS (HIP FLEXORS)

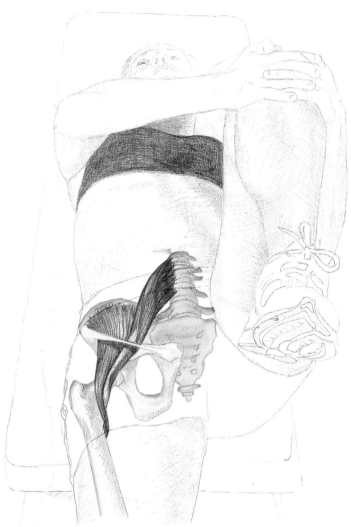

If there are any main culprits when it comes to causing lower-back problems, they would be the hip flexors. They have the strength and the position to wreak havoc. Anybody who works sitting down constantly shortens these muscles. Shortened muscles eventually make it impossible to either stand or walk without pain in the lower back. Many stretches for these muscles exist, but few are both effective and safe. If you make a mistake, you can create more pain instead.

MUSCLE FACTS

The psoas and the iliacus are situated deep in the muscular system, originating from the front side of the lower vertebrae and the front of the hip bone. They run down the front side of the pubic bone and attach to the inside of the upper femur. The psoas and the iliacus flex and internally rotate the hip joint, as well as increase the arch of the lower back.

Causes of Tightness

These muscles become shortened by any activity that flexes the hips for a long period of time, such as sitting. Working the hip flexors statically, as in doing sit-ups with poor technique, can also create tension.

Symptoms of Tightness

• Ache or pain in the lower back
• Pain in the groin or the inside of the thigh

Flexibility Test

Lie on your back with both knees bent and pulled up toward your rib cage. Grab one knee and pull it in further, carefully straightening the other leg and resting it on the floor. Do not allow the foot of the straightened leg to turn out to the side.

Precautions

Avoid this exercise if, during the stretch, you feel pinching in the groin or the bent leg, or if you have lower-back pain.

TECHNIQUE

Sit on the edge of a stable table or a bench. Lie down on your back and pull both your legs up toward your rib cage with your hands. At this point, your entire lower back should rest on the surface. Grab your left knee with both hands and carefully extend your right leg until it hangs freely in the air. If your left knee is still pulled toward your ribcage and your lower back is still resting on the surface, you have reached the starting point.

Stretch for 5 to 10 seconds by relaxing the hanging leg. Let it hang for 5 to 10 seconds. For an even greater stretch, hang a weight, such as a backpack with books in it, from your leg. You can also actively pull your leg down to simulate a weight. Next, relax the muscles for 5 to 10 seconds.

Resist by lifting your right leg toward the ceiling for 5 to 10 seconds.

Deepen the stretch by continuing to relax the hanging leg until you reach a new ending point. Let it hang for 10 to 20 seconds.

Repeat two or three times.

Common Mistakes
- Lying too far in on the table and restricting the motion of the hanging leg
- Lying too far out on the table and increasing the arch
- Failing to pull the leg far enough toward the rib cage

Comments
If you have pain in your lower back, check your starting position again. The most common mistake is failing to position the leg against the rib cage, which moves the lower back away from the surface.

Finding a place to do this stretch can sometimes be difficult. A kitchen table is a good choice. To ensure that the surface stays stable, make sure that you sit across the table diagonally rather than on the edge.

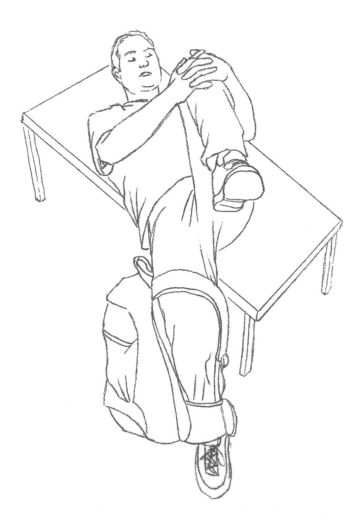

To increase the stretch in the muscle, you can hang a weight or a bag from your leg. Lying across the table diagonally decreases the risk of knocking it over.

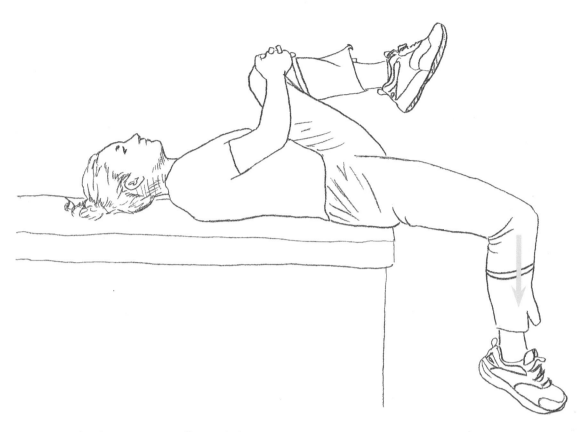

To protect your back, you must pull your left leg in toward your chest. Make sure to maintain contact between your lower back and the table at all times. Slowly lower your right leg without moving your left leg and relax.

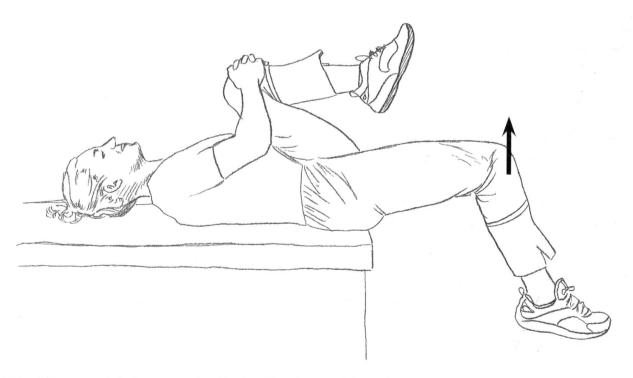

Resist by lifting your right leg a couple of inches (5 cm) toward the ceiling.

RECTUS FEMORIS (SUPINE VERSION)

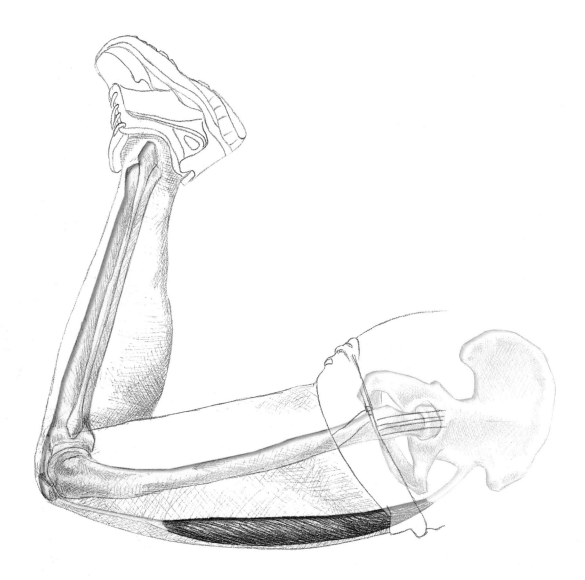

The rectus femoris is one of the four muscles that make up the group of muscles on the front of the thigh. It is the only one of these four muscles that runs across both the knee joint and the hip joint. This makes it special, since it can affect the lower back, the hip, and the knee joint.

Several bad options for stretching the front of the thigh exist. These stretches have led many people to believe that they are more flexible in this area than they might actually be. The worst stretch is pulling the heel up toward the buttocks while standing.

To do the following exercise, you will need a bench and a rope. Good, supportive shoes are also helpful if the floor is slippery.

MUSCLE FACTS

The rectus femoris originates from the front of the hip, runs across the hip and knee joints, and then attaches to the top front of the lower leg, joining with the other three muscles of the quadriceps group at the patellar tendon. The other three muscles are also stretched during this exercise; however, they do not have the same significance in terms of your well-being.

The rectus femoris extends the knee joint, bends the hip joint, and increases the arch of the lower back.

Causes of Tightness

The rectus femoris is shortened by daily sitting or through activities that work the muscle a lot, such as running, soccer, hockey, and biking.

Symptoms of Tightness

- Pain in the lower back
- Pain across and around the patella

Flexibility Test

Lie on your front with your forehead against the floor. Make sure that your knees are together and your abs are tight. Slowly bend your knees, keeping them together. You should be able to bend your knees to an angle of approximately 110 degrees without lifting your hips off the floor. You could also ask a partner to monitor whether the arch of your lower back increases before you reach 110 degrees.

Precautions

Avoid this exercise if you have pain in the lower back or the knee during the stretch.

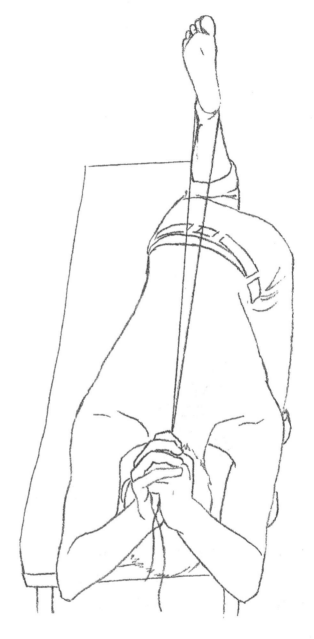

Make sure that you pull your heel straight toward your buttocks.

TECHNIQUE

Find a solid, flat surface. The height of the surface depends on your height and flexibility. The most important concern is that you do not arch your back at any point during the exercise. Put your right foot in the loop of a rope and run the rope across your right shoulder. Put your left foot on the floor in front of you and rest your body on top of the bench. Make sure that your entire left foot touches the floor and that your lower leg is perfectly vertical.

Bring your right leg, which is resting on the bench, slightly to the left. As long as your knee stays on the bench, you can allow the foot to move just beyond the

bench. If you have done this part correctly, your body should form the shape of a bow, creating a stretch that is more effective. Grab the rope above your head with both arms.

Stretch the muscle for 5 to 10 seconds by carefully straightening your arms so that the rope pulls on the foot. Pull until you feel a stretch on the front of your thigh. Relax the muscle for 5 to 10 seconds.

Resist by holding the rope steady and pushing your right knee into the bench while trying to straighten your right knee for 5 to 10 seconds. Relax for 5 to 10 seconds.

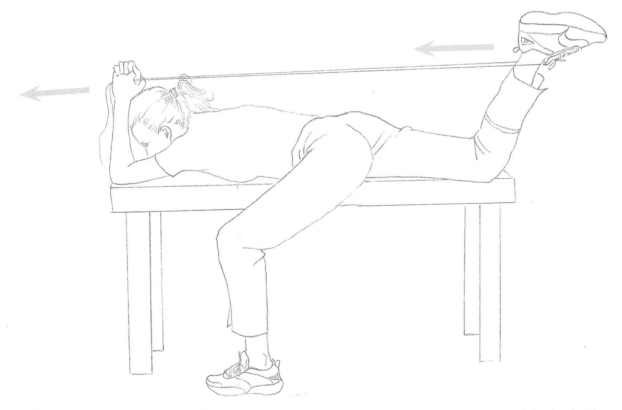

The left leg needs to be positioned far enough forward to prevent any change to the arch of the back. The height of the surface depends on your flexibility and height. Plant your left foot on the floor, tighten your abs, and carefully pull the rope.

Deepen the stretch by continuing to straighten your arms above your head until you reach another ending point.

Repeat two or three times.

Common Mistakes

- Using a bench that is too high
- Failing to position the left foot far enough forward
- Using a rope is too short

Comments

A bench that is too high creates an arch in the lower back, which defeats the purpose of the stretch. If your rope is too short, you cannot grip it above your head and you end up pulling your arm behind you. If you don't have access to a long rope, use a scarf or a couple of belts that are tied together.

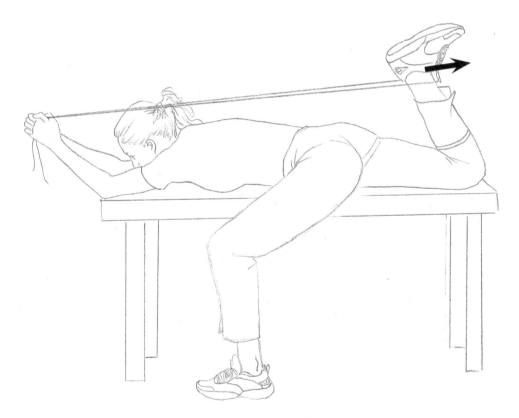

Resist by carefully pressing your right knee into the bench while straightening your leg.

RECTUS FEMORIS (KNEELING VERSION)

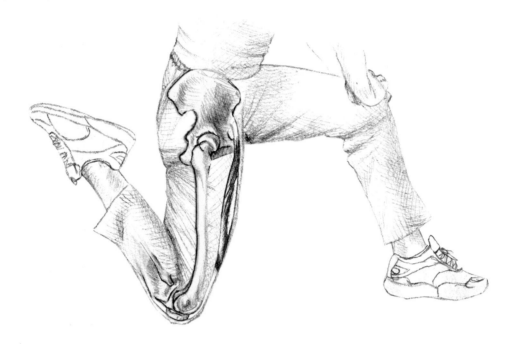

Try this variation if your hamstrings are too tight for the supine version. In this case, you have to consider that two joints are working together (the knee joint and the hip joint). The hip joint needs to be open and straight throughout the exercise. Keep your abs tight to prevent arching the lower back.

Precautions

Avoid this exercise if you have problems around your kneecaps.

TECHNIQUE

Kneel facing away from a wall. Your toes should touch the wall. Bring your left leg forward so that the entire foot touches the floor and your left shin is vertical. Lean your upper body forward and rest it on your left thigh. Let your right knee slide backward toward the wall and your right foot slide up the wall. Stop when your right knee is bent to 90 degrees. You have now reached the starting position.

Stretch the muscle for 5 to 10 seconds by carefully straightening your arms so that your upper body and thigh move closer to the wall. Stop when you feel a slight sting in the front of your thigh. Relax the muscle for 5 to 10 seconds.

Resist for 5 to 10 seconds by carefully pushing your right knee into the floor as you push your foot against the wall. Relax the muscle for 5 to 10 seconds.

Deepen the stretch by continuing to straighten your arms until you reach a new ending point. You can also use your right knee to carefully slide closer to the wall.

Repeat two or three times.

Common Mistakes

- Failing to tighten the abs and allowing the lower back to arch
- Flexing the hip joint, thereby lessening the stretch
- Positioning the knee too close to the wall, creating too much force and preventing a straight back
- Failing to flex the knee enough in the starting position
- Allowing the back foot to slide down the wall to the side

Comments

If your back hurts during or after this exercise, you might want to try the previous exercise for a while. If your knee hurts, try putting a pillow on the floor.

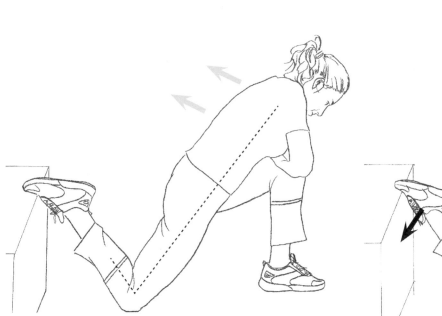

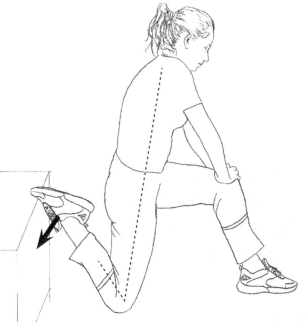

Your thigh and torso should be in a straight line. Tighten your abs and extend your arms. Avoid arching your back or bending your hip.

Resist by carefully straightening your leg.

TENSOR FASCIAE LATAE

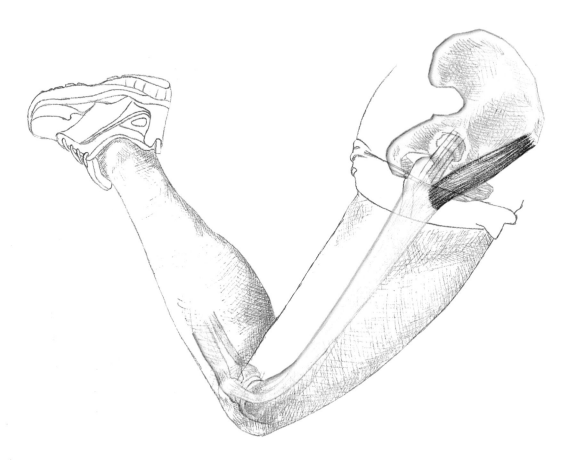

This exercise is similar to the kneeling one for the rectus femoris. However, in this exercise, the upper body and the leg form the shape of a bow. Remember to keep your abs tight to prevent arching the lower back or bending the hip.

MUSCLE FACTS

The tensor fasciae latae originates from the front of the outside of the hip, runs downward, and attaches to the outside of the thigh with a strong tendon. This tendon, the iliotibial tract, continues down past the outside of the knee before attaching to the upper part of the shinbone. The tensor fasciae latae flexes your hip and brings your leg out to the side. Since its tendon attaches below the knee, it also helps straighten the knee.

Causes of Tightness

Sitting for long periods of time, running, hiking, and biking can all shorten this muscle.

Symptoms of Tightness

- Pain on the outside of the hip (snapping hip) and thigh
- Pain on the outside of the knee (runner's knee) and around the kneecap
- Aching and pain in the lower back

Precautions

Avoid this exercise if you have pain in the lower back or knee during the stretch.

TECHNIQUE

The starting position is similar to the one used for stretching the rectus femoris. However, in this exercise, you will try to shape your upper body and leg like a bow. Kneel facing away from a wall with your toes touching the wall. Bring your left leg forward so that the entire foot touches the floor and your shin is vertical. Lean your body forward and rest it on your left thigh. Slide your right knee backward toward the wall and your right foot up along the wall. Stop when your knee is bent to 90 degrees.

Next, slide your foot along the wall 12 inches (30 cm) to the left. Tighten your abs and place your hands on your left knee. Bend your upper body to the left slightly, creating a bow with your leg. You have now reached the starting position.

Stretch for 5 to 10 seconds by slowly straightening your arms. Do not arch your lower back or bend your hip. Continue until you feel a sting on the outside of your thigh. Relax the muscle for 5 to 10 seconds.

Resist by carefully pushing your right knee into the floor as you push your foot against the wall. Relax the muscle for 5 to 10 seconds.

Deepen the stretch by continuing to straighten your arms without arching your back or flexing your hip until you reach a new ending point.

Repeat two or three times.

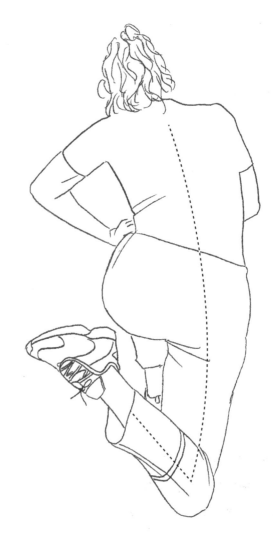

Your upper body and thigh should be in the shape of a bow, with your lower leg angled inward.

Common Mistakes

- Increasing the arch of the lower back instead of pushing the leg and upper body into a straight line
- Bending the hip, forcing it to shorten the muscle instead of stretching it
- Failing to assume the correct starting position with your leg and upper body shaped like a bow
- Failing to bend the knee enough

Comments

If you are not feeling a stretch in the muscle, your knee may be positioned too far from the wall. Decrease the angle at the starting position.

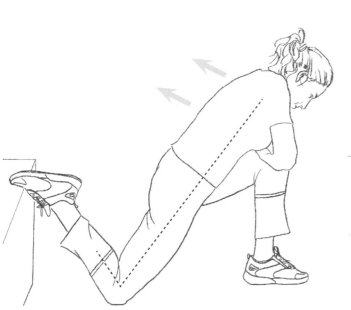

Your thigh and torso should be in a straight line. Tighten your abs and straighten your arms. Avoid arching your back or bending your hip.

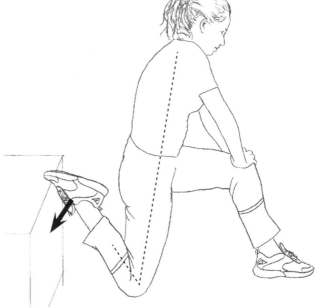

Resist by carefully straightening your leg.

HAMSTRINGS

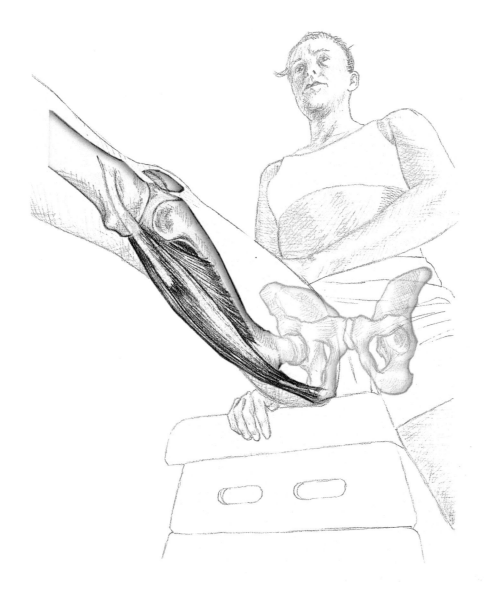

Two conditions must be present to achieve a good stretch on the back of the thigh. First, you have to arch your lower back a lot. If you curve the lower back, you decrease the stretch in the muscle. Second, your foot should not be on top of the bench, but should be outside the edge. If your foot is on the bench, you might be limited by the flexibility of your calves.

To take your calves out of the exercise further, point your toes. Remember that the leg that is off the bench is there to help you increase the arch of the lower back, thereby increasing the stretch in the hamstrings.

Make sure that your left leg is pulled as far back as possible.

MUSCLE FACTS

The muscles on the back of your thigh mainly consist of four separate muscles. Three of these originate from the sit bones on the hips and one originates from the back of the femur. All of them attach to the upper part of the lower leg. The hamstrings flex the knee joint, extend the hip, and tilt the hip backward, decreasing the arch in the lower back.

Causes of Tightness

The hamstrings can become shortened if you sit a lot or are generally inactive. Sports such as running, skiing, soccer, and hockey also shorten the hamstrings.

Symptoms of Tightness

• Ache or pain in the lower back
• Difficulty bending forward
• Shortened (less efficient) walking or running step
Tightness can increase the risk of cramping on the back side of the thigh.

Flexibility Test

Lie on your back, holding both legs completely straight. Raise one leg toward the ceiling until it is perpendicular to the floor. You should be able to reach a 90-degree angle in the hip.

Precautions

Avoid this exercise if you have pain in your back or around the kneecap during the stretch, or if you only feel the stretch in your Achilles tendon.

TECHNIQUE

Sit on a bench or something similar. Two chairs without armrests work well.

Sit so that your entire right leg rests on the surface. Make sure that your right foot is placed outside the edge. Put one hand under your knee to ensure that your right leg is slightly bent. Place your left foot as far back as possible (move until you feel a stretch on the front side of the thigh). Make sure that your left foot is planted on the floor.

Sitting up straight with tight abs, actively try to increase the arch in your lower back. Feel free to hold the bench with your hand.

You have now reached the starting position.

Stretch by slowly moving the upper body forward and down until you feel a slight sting on the back side of your thigh. Relax the muscles for 5 to 10 seconds.

Resist by carefully pushing your right leg into the bench for 5 to 10 seconds. Relax the muscles for 5 to 10 seconds.

Deepen the stretch by continuing to reach forward and down with your upper body until you reach a new ending point.

Repeat two or three times.

Common Mistakes

• Bending the back instead of the hip when stretching forward and down
• Increasing the bend in the knee while leaning forward
• Failing to position the passive leg far enough back

Comments

If you still feel a greater stretch in your calves than in the hamstrings, try bending the knee of the stretching leg more at the starting position.

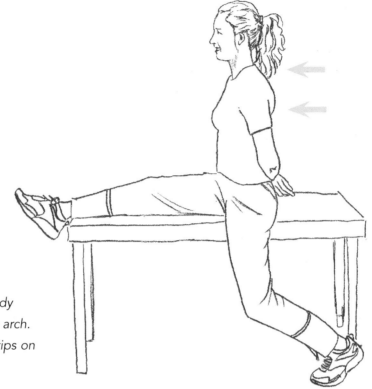

Place your left leg as far behind you as possible. Lift your upper body and tighten your abs. Lean your upper body forward while maintaining the arch. Feel free to place your fingertips on the bench for support.

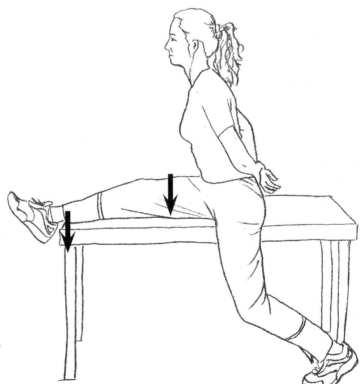

Resist by pressing your foot and thigh into the bench without moving your upper body.

PECTINEUS, ADDUCTOR LONGUS, AND ADDUCTOR BREVIS (SHORT ADDUCTORS)

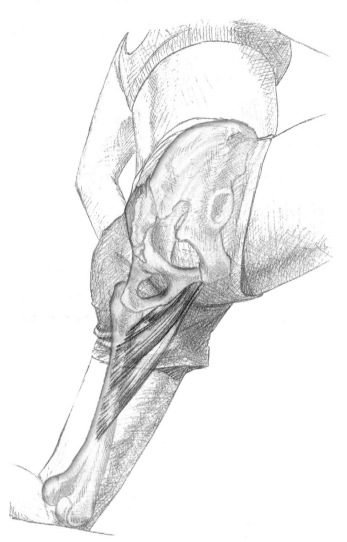

Since the muscles on the inside of the thigh are often quite sensitive, this easy warm-up exercise is recommended. It will help you locate the right muscles so that you can stretch them correctly. Your left leg controls this entire exercise, including how far you take the stretch. Make sure that your left leg does the work while your right leg relaxes. Sometimes this exercise is referred to as the Indian due to the placement of the legs in the starting position.

MUSCLE FACTS

The short adductors consist of three muscles. They originate from the front of the pubic bone, run down the inside of the thigh, and then attach to the back of the femur. The short adductors bring the legs toward each other and rotate the legs outward. They also help tilt the hips forward, increasing the arch of the lower back.

Causes of Tightness

Muscle tightness occurs if you sit too much or if you are generally inactive. These adductors can also be shortened by sports, such as hockey, soccer, and horseback riding.

Symptoms of Tightness

• Ache or pain in the lower back

The risk for pulling the groin muscles is greater if your adductors are tight.

Precautions

Avoid this exercise if you have pain in the knee or the lower back during the stretch.

Warm up before stretching the short adductors.

Since the muscles on the inside of the thigh can be somewhat sensitive, do this warm-up exercise before stretching them.

Stand in the starting position. Sway from side to side, using your right leg. Alternate using the inside of your thigh and your gluteal muscles.

Start stretching when you feel warmed up.

TECHNIQUE

Kneel on the floor. Bring your left leg out to the side and place your foot on the floor. Make sure that your right thigh and your left thigh form a right angle. Your left foot should point in the same direction as your left knee.

Make sure that your left knee is bent to form a right angle and your right hip is open. Tighten your abs and slightly decrease the arch in your lower back without bending your right hip. Your upper body should be completely upright.

This is your starting position.

Stretch for 5 to 10 seconds by carefully bending your left knee and pressing your right knee to the right until you feel a slight sting on the inside of your right thigh. Relax the muscle for 5 to 10 seconds.

Resist by carefully pressing your right knee to the left for 5 to 10 seconds. Relax the muscle for 5 to 10 seconds.

Deepen the stretch by continuing to bend the left knee and pressing the right knee to the right until you reach a new ending point.

Repeat two or three times.

Common Mistakes
- Flexing the hip joint
- Arching the lower back too much
- Placing the left foot too close to the body

Comments

As you become more flexible, place your left foot farther away in the starting position. Place a pillow under your knee if it hurts. Tighten up your abs if you feel any pain in your lower back.

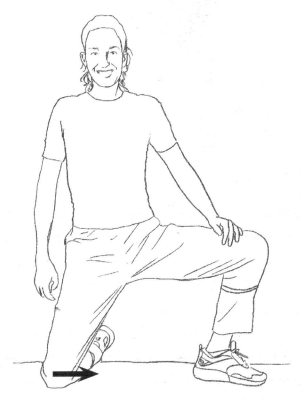

Lift your upper body and tighten your abs. Carefully bend your left leg to bring your left knee out to the side.

Resist by pressing your right knee to the left without actually moving your body.

GRACILIS
(LONG ADDUCTOR)

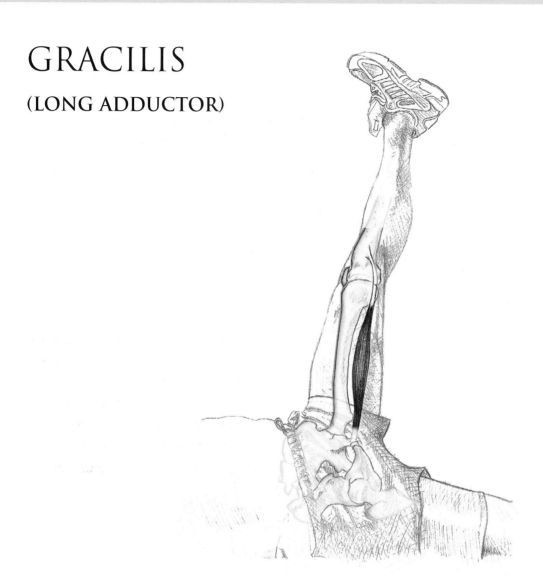

The gracilis affects both the knee and hip joints. If you want to achieve a good stretch in this muscle, you need to straighten your leg as you bring it to the side instead of bending your leg, as in the stretch for the short adductors. Using a straight leg does increase the risk of injury to the knee joint, so be careful when doing this exercise and avoid similar exercises done standing up. To be on the safe side, after finishing the stretch, bend your knee before you bring the leg back. It is a good idea to do the previous warm-up exercise before this exercise.

MUSCLE FACTS

The gracilis is a long, thin muscle that originates from the front of the pubic bone. It runs along the inside of the thigh by the inner knee and attaches to the inner and upper part of the lower leg. Occasionally, this muscle's tendon is used to surgically replace the anterior cruciate ligament (ACL) in the knee.

The gracilis flexes the hip and knee joints. It tilts the hips forward and increases the arch of the lower back.

Causes of Tightness

The gracilis will get tight if you sit a lot or if you are generally inactive. It can also be shortened by sports, such as hockey, soccer, and horseback riding.

Symptoms of Tightness

• Pain on the inside of the knee.

Precautions

Avoid this exercise if you have pain on the inside of the knee during the stretch.

TECHNIQUE

Lie on the floor to the right of a door frame with your buttocks placed against the wall and your legs running straight up it. Bend your left leg so that your thigh and knee rest against the inside of the door frame. This makes the exercise stable and protects your back. Your right leg should be completely straight as it points toward the ceiling. Tighten your abs and place your arms straight out to the sides.

Stretch for 5 to 10 seconds by very carefully moving your leg sideways along the wall. Slide your heel along the wall until you feel a sting on the inside of your thigh. Relax the muscle for 5 to 10 seconds.

Resist by carefully raising your leg along the wall about an inch (2.5 cm). Relax the muscle for 5 to 10 seconds.

Deepen the stretch by letting the leg slide out to the side until you reach a new ending point.

Repeat two or three times.

Common Mistakes

• Bending the right leg too much

• Failing to tighten the abs enough

• Positioning yourself too far from the wall

Comments

If you have sensitive adductors, you can start by doing the exercise for the short adductors on page 98. You can also simply do this exercise little by little. Bring your leg out to the side and then back to the starting position. Repeat the action, bringing the leg a little farther out to the side before bringing it back in. Move about 4 inches (10 cm) farther each time to warm up the muscle.

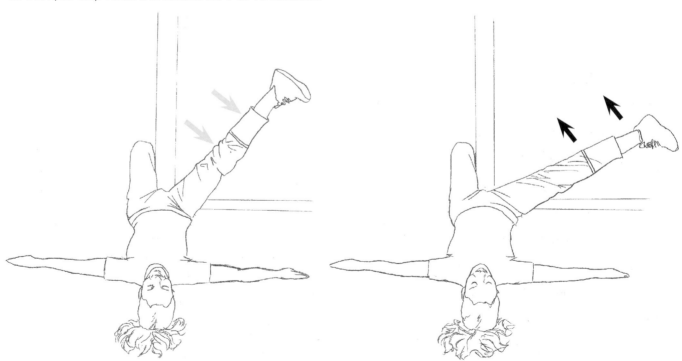

Lie as close to the wall as possible and place your left leg against the door frame. Carefully bring your right leg out to the side.

Resist by carefully pulling your right leg back up along the wall 1 to 2 inches (2.5 to 5 cm).

GASTROCNEMIUS

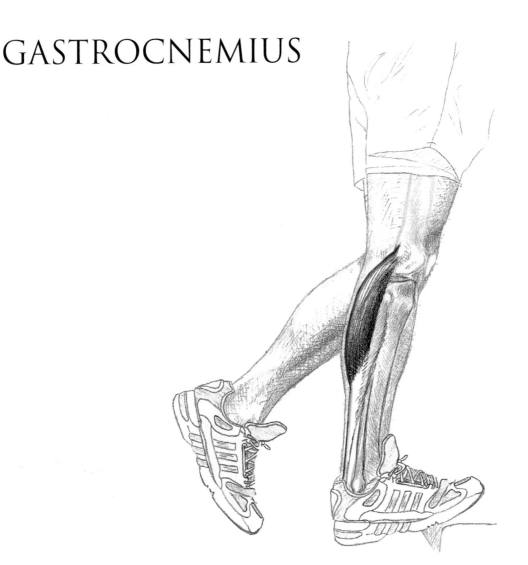

The gastrocnemius is one of the strongest muscles in the body. Despite its small size, it can easily lift the weight of the entire body. Running and jumping are two examples. The muscle and its tendons also have very strong endurance. They are created for long-lasting loads of low intensity, such as walking long distances. The muscle needs a lot of time and force to actually stretch out. For this reason, you should stretch for a full minute each time to get the desired result. Exercises in which you both stand and step will do almost nothing for this muscle. To get some variation in the stretching of this muscle, stand on a surface that leans a couple of degrees to the side. Always use shoes when doing this exercise.

MUSCLE FACTS

This large calf muscle has two heads that both originate from the back, lower part of the femur. They run together to form the Achilles tendon, which attaches to the heel. The gastrocnemius points the foot and bends the knee.

Causes of Tightness

The gastrocnemius may become tight from long periods of inactivity or from long-distance running.

Symptoms of Tightness

- Cramping in the muscle belly
- Pain in the Achilles tendon (possibly leading to Achilles tendonitis)
- Pain in the muscles on the front of the lower leg
- Pain in the arch of the foot

Precautions

Avoid this exercise if you have pain on the top of the foot.

TECHNIQUE

Find a steady edge, such as a step or a couple of phone books. Position your right foot so that the pad of the foot (about one-third of the foot) touches the surface and the arch and the heel are in the air.

Stretch by relaxing your calf and letting your heel drop down. Relax the muscle for 5 to 10 seconds.

Resist by using your calf muscles to raise your body 1 to 2 inches (2.5 to 5 cm). Relax the muscle for 5 to 10 seconds.

Deepen the stretch by dropping your heel down until you feel a slight sting in the muscle again. This is your new ending point.

Repeat two or three times.

Common Mistakes
- Standing too far over the edge
- Failing to straighten the leg

Comments

If it hurts to do this exercise, try stretching both calves at the same time.

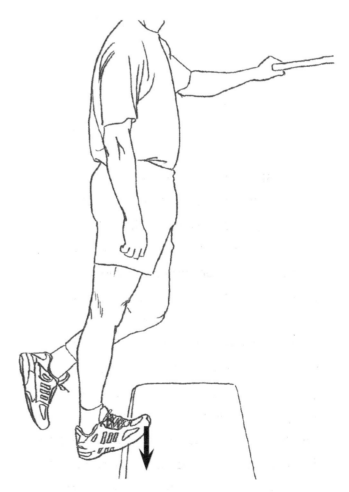

Stand with the ball of your foot on the surface. Make sure that your leg is completely straight. Carefully allow your heel to sink down.

Resist by pressing the ball of your foot against the surface.

SOLEUS

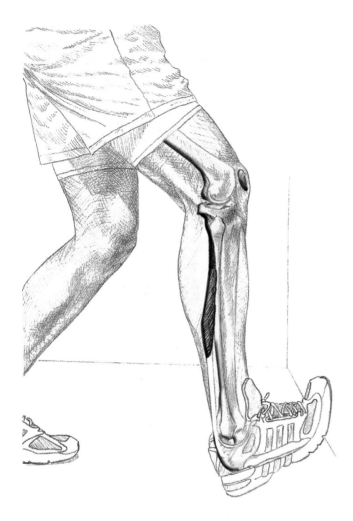

The difference between this deep-calf muscle and the gastrocnemius is that the soleus does not run past the knee joint. Therefore, it does not affect the knee joint. This exercise stretches the soleus without necessarily stretching the gastrocnemius. For this reason, you should keep your leg slightly bent when stretching the soleus.

MUSCLE FACTS

The soleus is located below the gastrocnemius. Both attach through the Achilles tendon. The soleus originates behind the bones in the lower leg and attaches to the heel. It also points the foot.

Causes of Tightness

The soleus tightens up during long periods of inactivity or habitual sitting. Sports that emphasize its use, such as running and biking, may also result in tension.

Symptoms of Tightness

- Ache or pain in the calf
- Ache or pain in the arch of the foot

A tight soleus can cause problems for the Achilles tendon as well.

Precautions

Avoid this exercise if it causes pain in the heel or in the back of the knee.

TECHNIQUE

Find a wall close to a door opening to help you maintain balance and increase the forward lean of your body. Put the ball of your right foot against the wall, keeping your heel on the ground. Use your back leg to make sure that you are stable. Carefully bend the right knee and grab the door frame. Tighten your abs and straighten your upper body. You are now in the starting position.

Stretch the muscle for 5 to 10 seconds by carefully leaning your leg and upper body forward, maintaining the angle of the knee, until you feel a slight sting in your calf. Relax the muscle for 5 to 10 seconds.

Resist by carefully pressing your foot into the wall, trying to point it, for 5 to 10 seconds. Relax the muscle for 5 to 10 seconds.

Deepen the stretch by continuing to lean your leg and upper body forward without straightening your knee until you reach a new ending point.

Repeat two or three times.

Common Mistakes
• Straightening the leg being stretched too much
• Positioning the ball of the foot either too high or too low on the wall

Comments
If you have pain in your heel during the stretch, be a little more careful or stretch the gastrocnemius for a while.

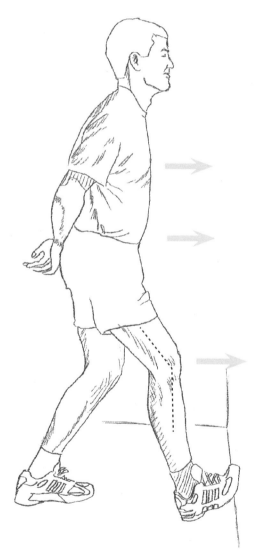

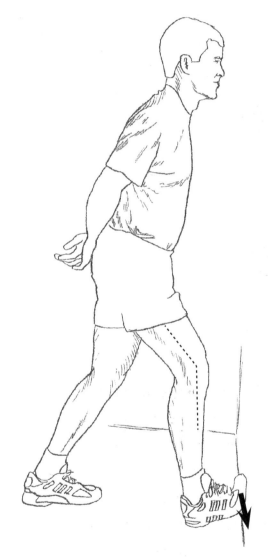

Make sure that your knee is bent during the entire exercise to prevent engaging the gastrocnemius. Feel free to use your arms to pull your body forward during the exercise.

Resist by pressing the ball of your foot into the surface without actually moving your body.

TIBIALIS ANTERIOR

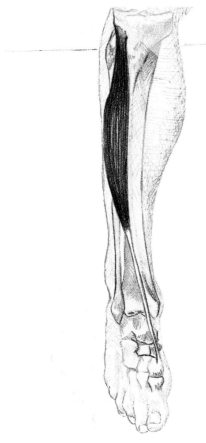

The tibialis anterior is difficult to stretch due to its position on the front of the shin and the limited mobility of the ankle joint. You will not feel the stretch in the muscle in the same way that you do when stretching other muscles. Other exercises, such as sitting on your heels, can provide a better stretch. The downside is the risk for injuring the knee joint. It is common to mistake overuse of the tibialis anterior for shin splints. Shin splints are usually found on the lower interior of the shinbone, rather than on the outside of the bone.

MUSCLE FACTS

The tibialis anterior is located on the front of the lower leg and the outside of the shinbone. It originates from the entire front side of the shinbone, runs across the ankle and the top of the foot, and attaches to the big toe. The tibialis anterior flexes the ankle and tilts the foot outward (supination).

Causes of Tightness

Tightness in the tibialis anterior may occur during fast walking if you are not used to it. The muscle may also tighten up while running or biking with clips on the pedals.

Symptoms of Tightness

- Ache or pain on the outside of the shinbone
- Ache or pain across the ankle
- Difficulty tilting the foot while walking or running because your ability to supinate the foot is limited.

Precautions

Avoid this exercise if you have pain in the ankle or the knee during the stretch.

TECHNIQUE

Find a soft surface that is somewhat higher than your knees. A tall bench or two pillows on a chair work well. Stand next to the bench and put your ankle on top of it. Place your right hand on your heel with your fingers facing forward to get a good grip.

Stretch for 5 to 10 seconds by pressing your heel forward and down with your hand until you feel a slight sting on the front of your ankle. Relax the muscle for 5 to 10 seconds.

Resist by pressing your toes down into the surface for 5 to 10 seconds. Relax the muscle for 5 to 10 seconds.

Deepen the stretch by pushing your heel forward and down until you reach a new ending point.

Repeat two or three times.

Common Mistakes

• Placing the bench or chair too low, making it hard to press the hand down

Comments

If you cannot achieve a good stretch in the muscle, ask a naprapath or a massage therapist to help you to relax.

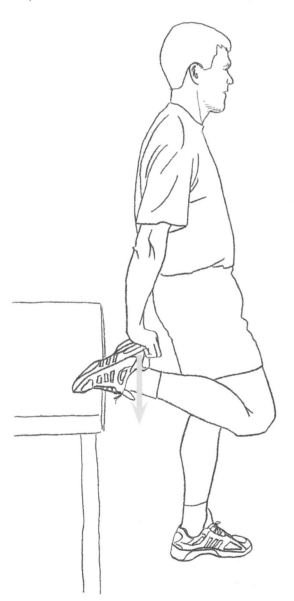

Avoid bending the knee too far. Push your heel down to extend your ankle while bending your right leg.

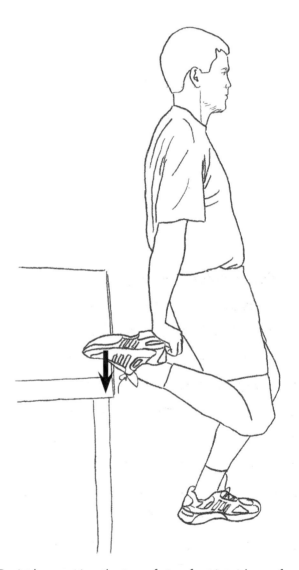

Resist by pressing the top of your foot into the surface.

BICEPS BRACHII

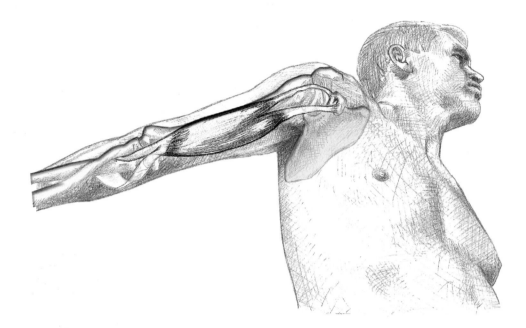

Since the biceps brachii runs past both the elbow and shoulder joints, it is important to be extra careful during this exercise. Although this stretch might not feel exactly like others, you can still benefit from it. Muscle tearing or rupture can be prevented by stretching.

MUSCLE FACTS

The biceps brachii is located on the front of the upper arm. It has two heads that originate in two separate places on the shoulder blade and come together to form one muscle belly on the middle of the upper arm. It attaches to the radius. The biceps brachii flexes the elbow and rotates the forearm externally (moving the palm of your hand to face up). It also helps bring the arms slightly out and forward in the shoulder joint.

Causes of Tightness

The biceps brachii can become tight and shortened during activities that keep the elbow in a flexed position, such as shoveling snow or carrying heavy objects.

Symptoms of Tightness

• Ache or pain on the front and outside of the shoulder
• Pain on the front of the elbow

Precautions

Avoid this exercise if you have pain in the wrist, elbow, or shoulder joint during the stretch.

TECHNIQUE

Find a ledge or a bar at or just below shoulder height, depending on your flexibility. Stand facing arm's length away from the ledge or bar. Your right arm should be rotated inward so that your thumb points toward your hip. Bring your arm backward in the same position and grab the bar or rest the back of your hand on the ledge. Your knuckles should now point downward and your thumb should point toward your body. Bring your body up, tighten your abs, and take a small step forward with your right leg. You have now reached the correct starting position.

Stretch for 5 to 10 seconds by carefully bending both legs without leaning your upper body forward. Continue until you feel a slight sting on the front of your upper arm. Relax the muscle for 5 to 10 seconds.

Resist by pressing your arm down toward the floor for 5 to 10 seconds. Relax the muscle for 5 to 10 seconds.

Deepen the stretch by continuing to bend your knees until you reach a new ending point.

Repeat two or three times.

Common Mistakes

• Rotating the arm in the wrong direction

• Placing the bar either too high or too low

• Bending the upper body or leaning it forward

Comments

It is common to have difficulty feeling a stretch in the muscle belly on the front of the upper arm. You may only feel a stretch in the shoulder joint or the elbow. As long as it does not cause discomfort, this exercise can still be beneficial to you. If you have wrist pain while holding the bar, try leaning your upper body slightly forward when you reach the stretching position to extend your wrist. Place a towel on the ledge or bar if your hand hurts.

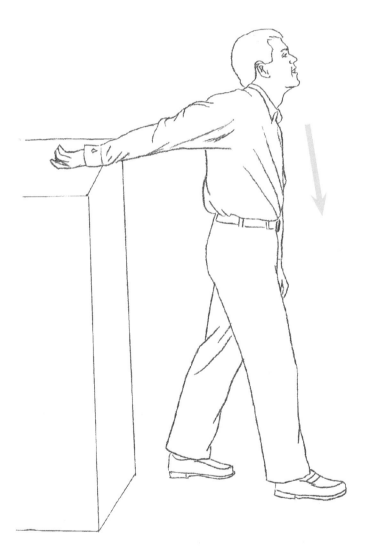

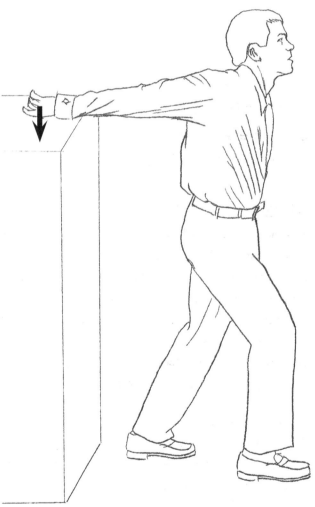

Rest the back of your hand on the surface. Grabbing a stationary pole will help you achieve a stretch that is even greater. Keep your upper body upright while you bend your legs.

Resist by pressing your hand down and forward.

TRICEPS BRACHII

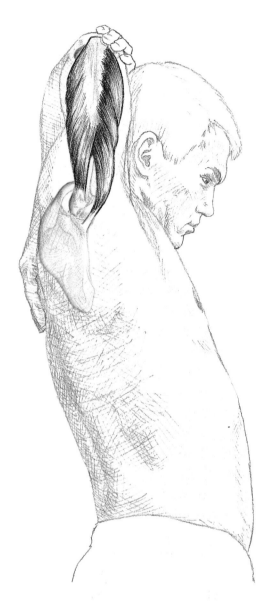

Although the muscles on the back of the upper arm are rarely injured, they can still cause different kinds of aches or pain. Trigger points or knots can cause radiating pain either down toward the elbow or up into the shoulder region. If you are very flexible in the shoulder joint, you should make sure that you anchor your shoulder blade against the wall.

MUSCLE FACTS

The triceps brachii, which is located on the back of the upper arm, has three heads that come together to form one muscle belly that attaches to the elbow. One of the heads originates from the shoulder blade and the other two originate from the back of the humerus. The triceps brachii straightens the elbow and brings the arm backward and slightly toward the body.

Causes of Tightness

The triceps brachii can become tight and shortened during sports such as tennis or badminton.

Symptoms of Tightness

• Ache or pain across the elbow

• Pain that radiates down the forearm

Precautions

Avoid this exercise if you have pain in the shoulder or the inside of the elbow during the stretch.

TECHNIQUE

Stand with your right side against a wall. Make sure that you are standing far enough from the wall so that you have to lean to reach it. Bring your right arm above your head so that only the shoulder blade touches the wall. Bend your right arm as far as you can. Grab your elbow with your left arm.

Stretch for 5 to 10 seconds by carefully pulling your right elbow behind your head until you feel a slight sting on the back of your upper arm. Relax the muscle for 5 to 10 seconds.

Deepen the stretch by continuing to bring your arm behind your head until you reach another ending point. You can increase the stretch by actively trying to bring your right elbow toward the ceiling.

Repeat two or three times.

Common Mistakes

- Tensing the chest, back, or shoulder
- Struggling to position the shoulder blade on the wall
- Failing to bend the elbow enough

Comments

Since this muscle is rarely severely shortened, most people will not feel a real stretch.

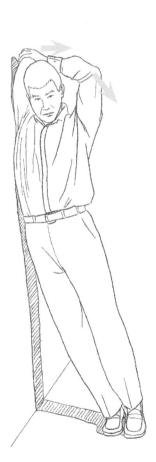
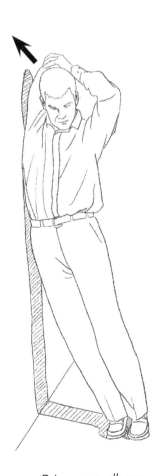
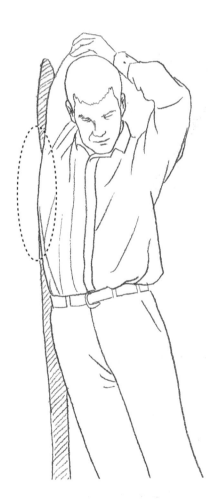

Bend your arm as much as you can. Bring your elbow behind your head to increase the stretch. Resist by bringing your elbow to the right while trying to straighten your arm.

Make sure that your shoulder blade is anchored against the wall.

FOREARM FLEXORS

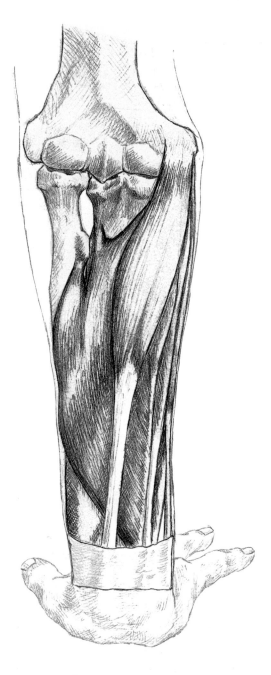

This section refers to the 10 small muscles in the forearm that are located on the same side as the palm of your hand. To avoid ache in these flexor muscles, you should stretch them often and avoid static and repetitive use over the long term.

MUSCLE FACTS

The flexors originate from the lower end of the upper arm and then run across the inside of the elbow joint and past the wrist on the palm side of the hand. Finally, they run out to the fingers in the form of tendons.

These flexors work as a group to bend the fingers toward the palm. They also work individually to bend each finger in its joint.

Causes of Tightness

These flexor muscles can become tight and shortened from extended static work such as operating a keyboard. Any occupation that requires extensive use of the hands can also cause problems for these muscles. Carpenters, massage therapists, naprapaths, gymnasts, climbers, and hockey players are often affected.

Symptoms of Tightness

• Pain and aching in the forearm and the fingers
• Pain on the inside of the elbow (also called golfer's elbow)

Flexibility Test

Bring your hand up in front of your face and put your palms together. Lift your elbows up and out until your forearms are horizontal. Do not move your hands.

Precautions

Avoid this exercise if it causes wrist pain.

TECHNIQUE

Find a flat surface, such as a table. Rotate your hands internally so that your fingers face toward you and place your hands on the table. Your right thumb should now point to the right.

Place your left hand over the fingers of your right hand. Straighten your right arm completely.

Stretch for 5 to 10 seconds by carefully pulling your right arm toward you until you feel a slight sting in your right forearm.

Relax your muscles for 5 to 10 seconds.

Resist by trying to push your fingers into the table for 5 to 10 seconds. Relax the muscles for 5 to 10 seconds.

Deepen the stretch by continuing to move your right arm toward you until you reach a new ending point.

Repeat two or three times.

Common Mistakes
- Bending the elbow
- Failing to keep the fingers completely straight
- Positioning the table too high

Comments
If the table is too high, it prevents the correct starting position and technique throughout the exercise. Placing your hand on a towel makes it easier to keep your fingers straight.

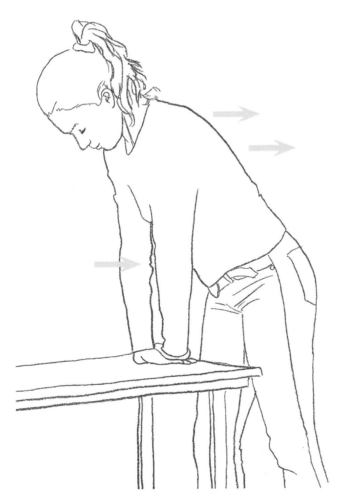

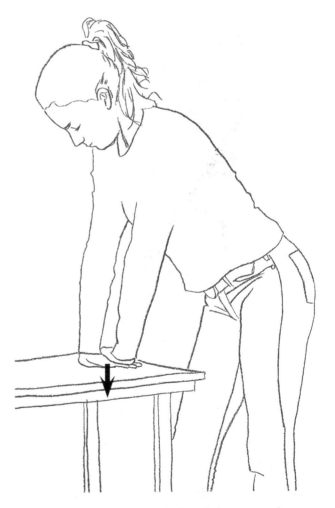

Lean your arm and body backward. Make sure that your elbow is completely straight during the exercise. Place your left hand over the fingers of your right hand to increase the stretch.

Resist by pressing your right hand down into the table.

FOREARM EXTENSORS

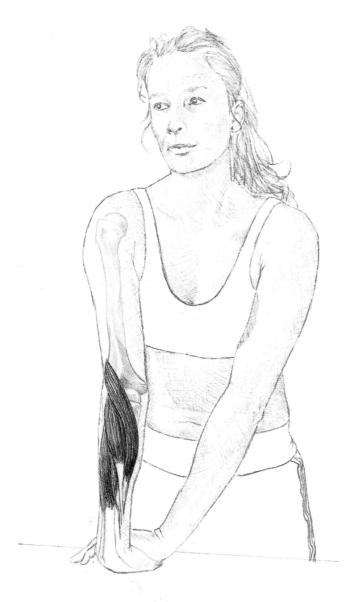

The extensors consist of 10 muscles which are located on the outside and back of the forearm. They have received a lot of attention lately because many people have been on sick leave due to aches and pain in this area. Stretch these muscles up to 20 times per day. In addition to providing the benefits of exercise, these stretches can be a good way to take a short break during work.

MUSCLE FACTS

Most of the extensors originate from the outside of the lower end of the upper arm. They run down the outside of the elbow and across the wrist, continuing down the hand and fingers as tendons. The extensors bend the elbow and flex the wrist toward the back of the hand. They also work individually to extend each finger in its joint.

Causes of Tightness

The extensors can become shortened by static work on the computer or by fine mechanical work. People who work mostly with their hands, such as carpenters, massage therapists, climbers, gymnasts, and weight lifters, are often affected.

Symptoms of Tightness

- Aching or pain in the forearms
- Aching or pain on the outside of the elbow (tennis elbow)
- Aching or pain in the fingers

Precautions

Avoid this exercise if it causes wrist pain.

TECHNIQUE

Use a table if you prefer to stand or use the floor if you prefer to sit. With the back of your hand facing forward, make a tight fist. Flex your wrist so that the back of your hand touches the table or floor and your fingers are facing you. Use your other hand to make sure that the fist is tight. Keep your elbow straight.

Stretch for 5 to 10 seconds by pulling your arm toward you until you feel a slight sting in the forearm. Relax the muscles for 5 to 10 seconds.

Resist by carefully pressing your knuckles into the table for 5 to 10 seconds. Relax the muscles for 5 to 10 seconds.

Deepen the stretch by continuing to pull your arm backward until you reach a new ending point.

Repeat two or three times

Common Mistakes
- Bending the elbow
- Failing to tighten the fist enough
- Positioning the table too high

Comments

If the table it too high, it prevents the correct starting position and technique throughout the exercise. Place a towel or a pillow on the table or the floor if the exercise hurts your hand.

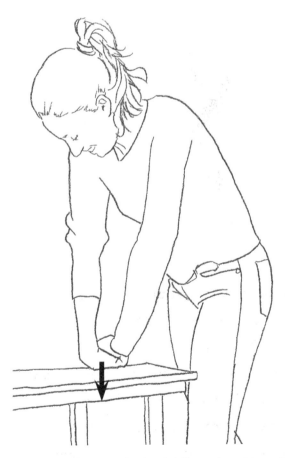

Use your left hand to keep the right fist closed and the fingers flexed. Make sure that your elbow is completely straight during the exercise. Pull your arm and body backward.

Resist by pressing the back of your hand into the table.

EXTENSOR CARPI RADIALIS LONGUS AND BREVIS

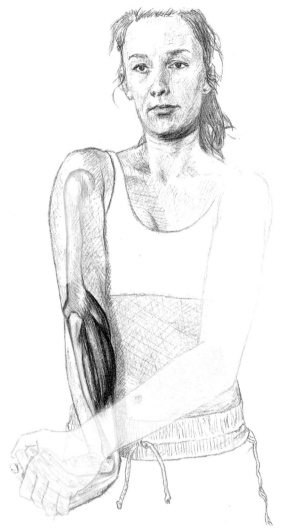

The extensor carpi radialis longus and brevis are the muscles that most often cause pain in the forearms due to static work with a computer mouse. These muscles can handle a lot of work, but year after year of the same work without a break will cause them to give out. Although we often do not want to listen, aches and pains are the muscles' way of protesting. Relieving pain in your forearms requires consistent stretching and thorough soft-tissue manipulation or massage.

The condition that took years to develop will also take a while to disappear. This kind of problem needs a long-term plan in order to improve.

MUSCLE FACTS

The extensor carpi radialis longus and brevis originate from the lower end of the upper arm and then run down past the elbow, along the outside of the forearm, and across the wrist. Finally, they attach to the index and ring fingers. These muscles bend the elbow and straighten the wrist, the index finger, and the ring finger.

Causes of Tightness

Long-term static work causes the extensor carpi radialis longus and brevis to shorten. People who work with their hands, such as construction workers, climbers, hockey players, and people who work with computers, are often affected.

Symptoms of Tightness

- Pain on the outside of the forearm
- Pain and numbness in the index and ring fingers
- Pain on the outside of the elbow (tennis elbow)

Precautions

Avoid this exercise if it causes pain in the wrist or in the shoulder.

TECHNIQUE

Bend your right arm and hold it in front of your navel. Make a fist and rotate your forearm inward as you flex your wrist in the direction of your palm. Grab the right fist with your left hand to flex the wrist more. Your elbow should remain bent. Relax your shoulder and right arm.

Stretch for 5 to 10 seconds by carefully extending your right arm while rotating your forearm inward, using your left hand to further flex the wrist. Continue until you feel a slight sting in your right forearm. Relax the muscles for 5 to 10 seconds.

Resist by carefully trying to straighten your right wrist for 5 to 10 seconds. Relax the muscles for 5 to 10 seconds.

Deepen the stretch by straightening your right arm and flexing your right wrist until you reach a new ending point.

Repeat two or three times.

Common Mistakes
- Failing to rotate the forearm enough
- Failing to flex the wrist enough
- Failing to tighten the fist enough
- Failing to straighten the right arm enough

Comments
Although this exercise can be a little tricky in the beginning, do not give up. Remember that practice makes perfect.

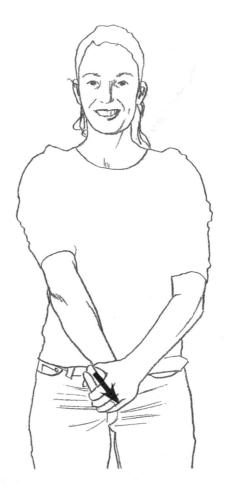

Bend your right arm and allow your left hand to flex the wrist and fingers. Straighten your arm and allow your left hand to keep the wrist and fingers in the same position.

Resist by pressing the back of your right hand against your left hand.

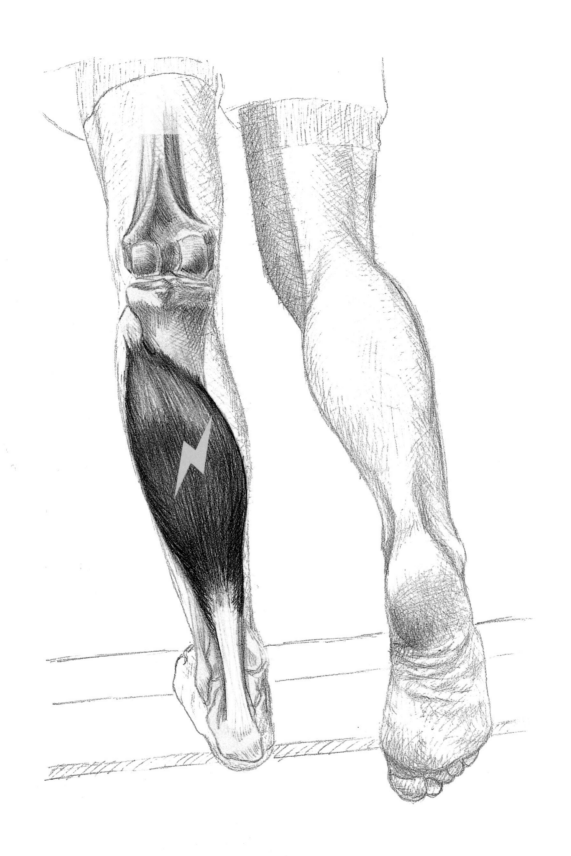

PROGRAMS
FOR PAIN RELIEF

COMMON MORNING ACHES AND PAINS

If it feels as if somebody has hit you over the head with baseball bat, tried to break your back, or pinned your arm behind your back during the night, your sleeping posture is probably working against you. Changing your sleeping position is not easy. You established this habit when you were young and your muscles are not as flexible now as they were back then. The following section suggests some remedies for pain commonly felt when waking.

DO YOU WAKE UP WITH A HEADACHE?

Waking up with a headache is far from the ideal way to start your day. Although you have been sleeping, you may not have been resting and relaxing. Grinding your teeth and clenching your jaw during sleep are typical symptoms of stress. This kind of nightly activity involves both the muscles in your jaw and the muscles in your neck. Have you have noticed that you want to pull your shoulder up toward your ear as you prepare to fall asleep? This action does not necessarily stop after you fall asleep, which may lead to a morning headache.

Remedies

Stretching and relaxing the area around the neck (see page 123) are very good ways to avoid headaches.

Headaches can be caused by poor sleeping posture combined with shortened muscles. The firmness of your bed may also be a factor. Generally speaking, the heavier you are, the firmer your bed should be.

DO YOU WAKE UP WITH A STIFF NECK?

If you wake up with a stiff neck that is hard to move, your pillow may be too tall. Sleeping on your side with a pillow that is too high stretches the muscles on one side of the neck and shortens the muscles on the other. This habit irritates the muscles and joints in the neck.

Remedies

Make sure that your head is aligned with your spine when you lie on your side. Adjust the height of your pillow as needed.

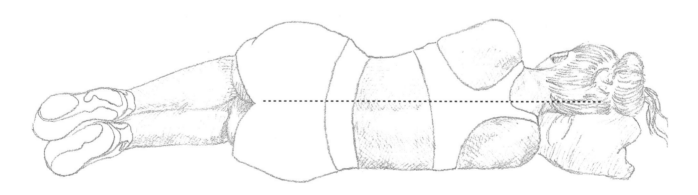

If you sleep on your side, make sure that your bed is not too soft. A firmer mattress may help maintain the alignment of the spine.

ARE YOUR ARMS ASLEEP WHEN YOU WAKE UP?

Experiencing numbness or tingling when you wake up can be uncomfortable. The most common reason for this is falling asleep with your arms above your head. Sleeping on your back with your arms above your head stretches the pectoralis major and minor, causing them to push on the nerves and blood vessels that run from the neck and trunk into your arms, which then fall asleep.

Remedies

Completely change your sleeping position or try sleeping with your arms by your sides. Stretch the pectoralis major and minor every night before you go to bed.

DOES YOUR SHOULDER HURT WHEN YOU WAKE UP?

Morning pain in the shoulder can be caused by sleeping with your arm under the pillow and your elbow above your head. Sleeping in this position squeezes the supraspinatus, which creates a feeling of weakness in the arm.

Remedies

Try sleeping on your back or keeping your arm below the shoulder.

DOES YOUR LOWER BACK HURT WHEN YOU WAKE UP?

Sleeping on your front in a bed that is too soft commonly results in the feeling that your back is breaking in two.

This is because your midsection, which is your heaviest part of the body, sinks down into the bed, severely arching your back. This habit, combined with tight hip flexors, almost guarantees lower-back pain in the morning.

Remedies

Switch to a firmer bed or place a board under the mattress. Stretch your hip flexors before you go to bed. Try sleeping on your side instead.

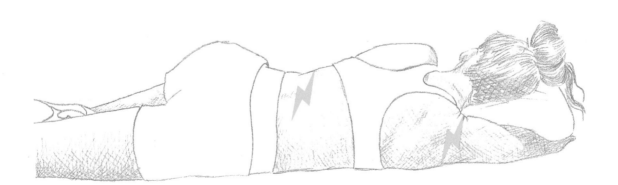

Any sleeping position that places the arms above the head can cause pain or numbness in the shoulder and arm. If you sleep on your front or in a bed that is too soft, you will increase the arch of your lower back, resulting in a slow back sprain.

STRETCHING SCHEDULE

Stretching is one of the best ways to eliminate or lessen pain. The rest of this chapter outlines stretching schedules for painful situations. When the text refers to throwing your back out or having a kink in your neck, reasons for the pain other than the ones mentioned may exist. If you are unsure of the reasons for your pain, seek the help of a physician or naprapath.

THROWING YOUR BACK OUT

This common expression does not really tell us anything about the reasons for the pain or what actually hurts.

What Hurts?

- Muscle spasms
- Stretched ligaments
- Injured discs
- Joint restriction in the lumbar spine

Background

Pain can be caused by the following:

- Muscular imbalance
- Fatigue in the back muscles
- Tight muscles
- Weak muscles
- Repeated heavy lifting
- General inactivity

General Remedies

The best suggestion is to keep moving. If possible, move your body from side to side in a range that feels safe. It doesn't matter how far you move your body as long as you move.

No matter how much it hurts, you need to get up and walk. Walk for as long as you can. If you get tired, lie down and rest. Make sure to lie on your side, since it is easier to get up from this position than from your front or your back. Avoid sitting down, which extends the healing process. Also avoid movements that send shooting pains to the limbs, since these trigger defense systems in your body, further prolonging the healing time.

Specific Remedies

Stretch several times every day. Stretching 10 times per day will help you feel better sooner.

When to Seek Professional Help

See a professional if you have any of the following:

- Shooting pain running down your leg
- Loss of sensitivity in certain parts of the skin
- Loss of strength in certain muscles
- Inability to urinate

Muscles to Stretch

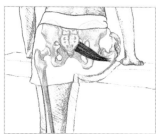

Piriformis, pages 72, 75

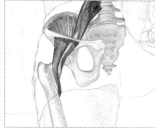

Psoas and iliacus, page 83

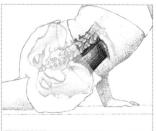

Quadratus lumborum, pages 78, 81

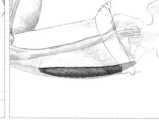

Rectus femoris, pages 86, 90

KINK IN YOUR NECK

This is another common expression that fails to tell us what has happened or what hurts. Movement is also key for this case, even if it hurts.

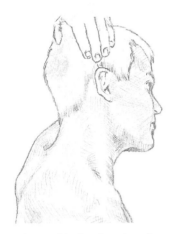

In general, two kinds of neck pain exist:

1. Type 1 occurs instantly. You cannot turn your head or tilt it to one side. The other direction is fairly painless. This kind of pain usually occurs right when you wake up in the morning.
2. Type 2 is a slow growing pain that decreases your mobility.

What Hurts?
- Muscle spasms
- Pinched nerves
- Compressed discs
- Stretched ligaments
- Joint restriction in the cervical spine

Background

Pain can be caused by the following:
- Overall tightness from stress or monotonous work
- Bad sleeping posture
- Acutely overloaded muscles
- Sitting in a drafty place

General Remedies

Movement is once again the key. If you are able, tilt and turn your head, moving it forward and backward. Stop the movement before you have pain. Avoid any neck braces and ice, but feel free to use heat. A grain pillow usually works very well.

Specific Remedies

Type 1. In the first case, only stretch in the direction that does not cause any pain.

Type 2. In the second case, stretch in both directions, but spend more time on the side in which mobility is limited.

For both kinds, it is important to stretch often. Stretching several times per hour is recommended.

When to Seek Professional Help

See a professional if you have any of the following:
- Shooting pain running from the neck into the arm and hand
- Loss of strength in the arm and hand
- Loss of sensitivity in certain areas of the skin

Muscles to Stretch

In addition to your own stretching, consider the help of a professional therapist, such as a naprapath, physical therapist, or chiropractor.

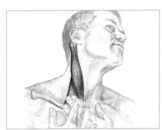
Sternocleidomastoid, page 30

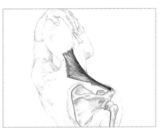
Upper trapezius, page 26

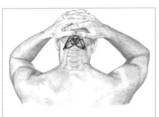
Suboccipitals, page 34

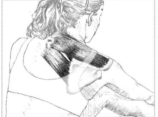
Middle trapezius and rhomboids, pages 48, 50

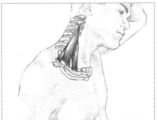
Scalenes, page 32

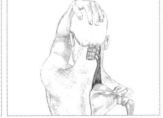
Levator scapulae, pages 36, 38

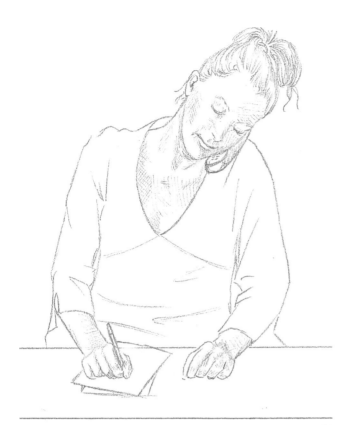

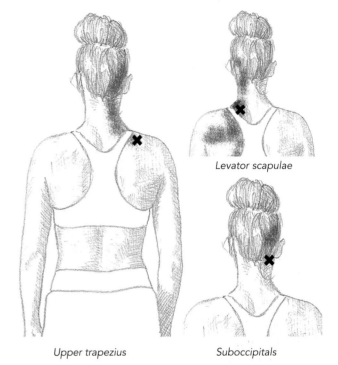

Levator scapulae

Upper trapezius

Suboccipitals

The actual amount of force on your spine is not necessarily the deciding factor for back or neck pain. Rather, the crucial variables are the position of the spine and the length of time the spine is in a specific position.

HEADACHE

Tension headache is the most common form of this kind of pain. Tight muscles in the neck and shoulders cause trigger points, which in turn lead to pain that runs up into your head. Common locations include on one side of the neck, past the temple, and behind the ear, where it may feel as if a nail is being driven in. This kind of pain almost always comes from a trigger point in the upper part of the trapezius. Therefore, massaging the temples will do nothing to relieve the pain. Since one headache can lead to more, stretching will help both temporarily and in the long run.

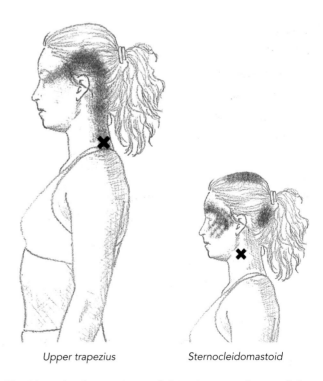

Upper trapezius

Sternocleidomastoid

The X marks the position of the trigger point, and the colored area indicates the possible spread of discomfort.

What Hurts?

- Trigger points
- Tight muscles
- Immobilized neck joints

Background

Pain can be caused by the following:

- Long-term tension from stress
- Monotonous work
- Worrying
- Pain in the shoulder region or in other parts of the body

General Remedies

It is important that you relax. When you feel a headache coming on, you may be able to stop it if you sit down right away, support your neck and shoulders, and then actively relax the neck and shoulders. A heating pad can also help relieve the tension.

Specific Remedies

Stretch the muscles mentioned in the following section. If your headache is too painful, actively rest and relax, then stretch when you feel a little better.

When to Seek Professional Help

See a professional if you have any of the following:

- Nonstop headache
- The headache becomes acute (exploding type), goes on nonstop, or you normally never have any headache at all.

Muscles to Stretch

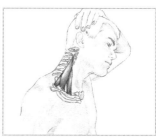

Upper trapezius, page 26

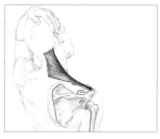

Scalenes, page 32

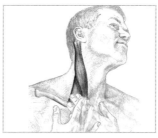

Sternocleidomastoid, page 30

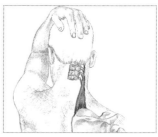

Levator scapulae, pages 36, 38

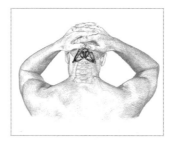

Suboccipitals, page 34

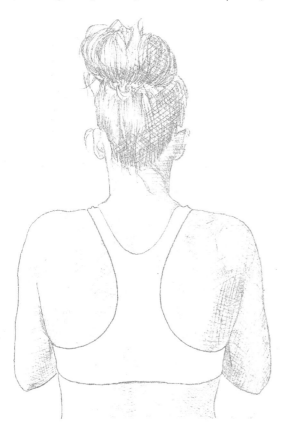

Continually sitting with your shoulders lifted is the most common reason for headache. To minimize your headache, practice relaxing and lowering your shoulders.

UPPER-BACK PAIN

It is not uncommon to have pain in one or more points in the upper back. The point inside of the upper part of the shoulder blade, which sometimes feels as if it is located under the shoulder blade, can be especially persistent. To get rid of the pain, you should stretch the muscles of the upper back, the chest, and the front of the neck. Without stretching the chest muscles, it is very difficult to improve your posture, which helps prevent pain.

What Hurts?
• Trigger points in the muscles
• Immobilized joints in the spine near the chest
• Immobilized joints between the ribs and the spine
• Overstretched ligaments

Background
Pain can be caused by the following:
• Bad posture
• Tight muscles in the chest, buttocks, and hamstrings
• Weak back muscles

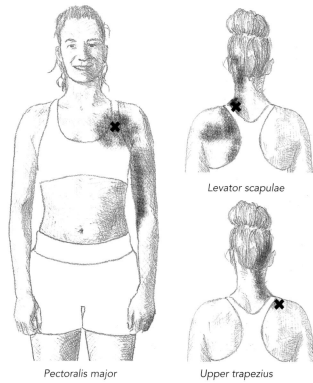

Levator scapulae

Pectoralis major   *Upper trapezius*

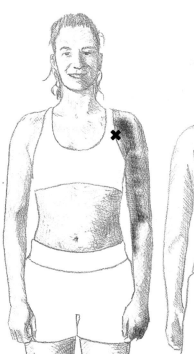
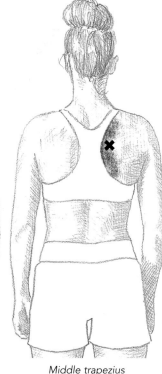

Pectoralis minor   *Middle trapezius*
                            Rhomboids

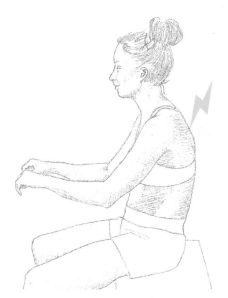

Hunching over while sitting forces the muscles between your shoulder blades to work statically in order to keep the body up and to protect the ligaments of the spine.

The X marks the position of the trigger point, and the colored area indicates the possible spread of discomfort.

General Remedies

The most important thing is to improve your posture. If you must sit, try not to do so for more than 20 minutes at a time. Stand up and move your shoulders, neck, and head if the muscles feel tight, even if you have only been sitting for five minutes. Try using a heating pad.

Specific Remedies

Take frequent, short breaks to stretch. These muscles will not give in easily.

When to Seek Professional Help

See a professional if the pain remains for a full week.

Muscles to Stretch

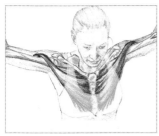

Pectoralis major, pages 40, 42

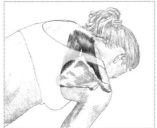

Middle trapezius and rhomboids, pages 48, 50

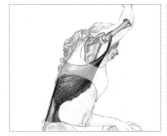

Latissimus dorsi, pages 52, 55

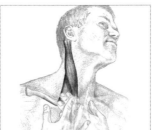

Sternocleidomastoid, page 30

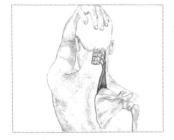

Levator scapulae, pages 36, 38

SHOULDER PAIN THAT RADIATES INTO THE ARM AND HAND

If you do not do a good job stretching your shoulder region, you increase your risk for pain that radiates into the arm and hand. For this reason, you should always stretch the muscles around the shoulder girdle first, followed by specific shoulder muscles and the arm muscles.

What Hurts?

• Trigger points in tight muscles
• Forearm muscles that are statically overloaded
• Joint restriction in the cervical spine

Background

Pain can be caused by small fine motor skills performed with the hand and forearm, which cause muscles in your shoulders to work statically just as much as the muscles in the forearm.

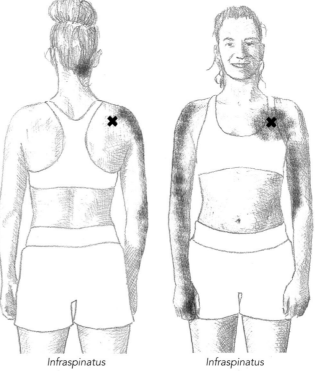

Infraspinatus

Infraspinatus
Pectoralis major

The X marks the position of the trigger point, and the colored area indicates the possible spread of discomfort.

Supraspinatus

Supraspinatus

Scalenes

Scalenes

The X marks the position of the trigger point, and the colored area indicates the possible spread of discomfort.

General Remedies

Examine everything you use in conjunction with the computer, such as your keyboard, the mouse, the height of the desk, and the chair. Get out of your chair every 20 minutes and move your shoulders around. When you are at home, try to unload these muscles and avoid static work of the shoulders and arms.

Specific Remedies

Stretch regularly, not just during your work hours.

When to Seek Professional Help

See a professional if the ache does not subside in three or four weeks.

Muscles to Stretch

First, stretch the muscles in the neck and around the shoulder girdle.

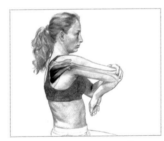
Infraspinatus, pages 57, 60

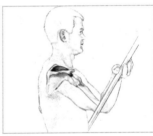
Supraspinatus, pages 64, 66

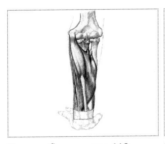
Forearm flexors, page 112

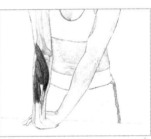
Forearm extensors, page 114

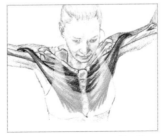
Pectoralis major, pages 40, 42

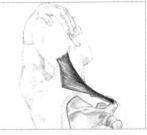
Upper trapezius, page 26

SHOULDER PAIN

Naturally, there are several reasons why your shoulder or the area surrounding it might hurt. Sometimes pain prevents the performance of any exercise. If this is the case for you, do not force yourself to stretch.

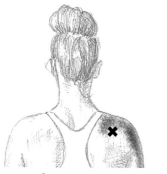
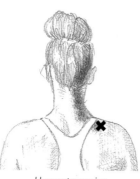

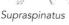
Supraspinatus   *Upper trapezius*

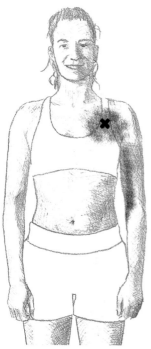
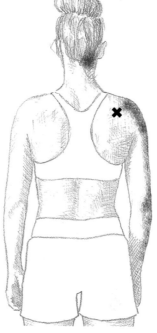

Pectoralis major   *Infraspinatus*

The X marks the position of the trigger point, and the colored area indicates the possible spread of discomfort.

What Hurts?
- Trigger points in tight muscles
- Pinched muscles
- Pinched nerves
- Joint cartilage damaged by injury
- Joints in the neck locking up

Background
Pain can be caused by the following:
- Repeated movements that rotate the shoulder joint either inward or outward
- Working a lot with your hands above your head
- Active participation in a throwing sport

General Remedies
Avoid all movements above the head and repeated rotation of the shoulder joint.

Specific Remedies
Stretch carefully, stopping if you feel pain.

When to Seek Professional Help
See a professional if you have any of the following:
- Nonstop pain
- Inability to complete shoulder movements due to pain or sudden resistance

Muscles to Stretch

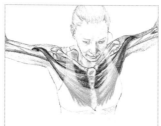
Pectoralis major, pages 40, 42

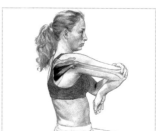
Infraspinatus, pages 57, 60

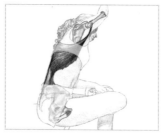
Latissimus dorsi, pages 52, 55

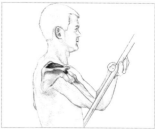
Supraspinatus, pages 64, 66

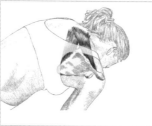
Middle trapezius and rhomboids, pages 48, 50

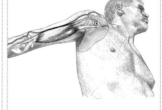
Biceps brachii, page 108

TENNIS ELBOW AND GOLFER'S ELBOW

These terms describe conditions that cause forearm pain. They are getting more and more common. Construction workers are often affected.

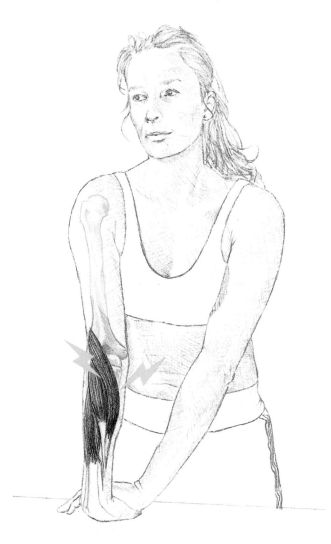

Golfer's elbow causes pain inside of the elbow, and tennis elbow causes pain on the outside.

What Hurts?

- Forearm muscles with overloaded attachments and a high concentration of lactic acid

Background

Pain can be caused by the following:

- Long-term static work using the forearms
- Work demanding strength endurance from both the forearms and the hands

General Remedies

Avoid all work with the forearms, including lighter tasks. Use a heating pad to increase the circulation in the forearms.

Specific Remedies

Stretch relentlessly, as often as 20 times per day.

When to Seek Professional Help

See a professional if you have pain that lasts longer than a week.

Muscles to Stretch

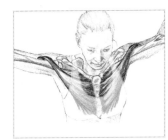
Pectoralis major, pages 40, 42

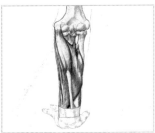
Forearm flexors, page 112

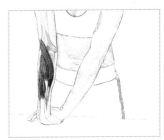
Forearm extensors, page 114

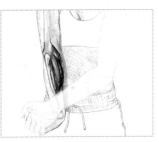
Extensor carpi radialis longus and brevis, page 116

RUNNER'S KNEE

Runner's knee is a common athletic injury that often affects people who do not exercise.

What Hurts?

• A short tendon fascia that originates at the tensor fasciae latae and gluteus medius and runs across the outside of the knee.

Background

Pain can be caused by the following:

• Tight and shortened muscles in the buttocks and thigh tighten up the fascia, causing it to rub against the outside of the knee

• Running, walking, or biking with an incorrect foot angle

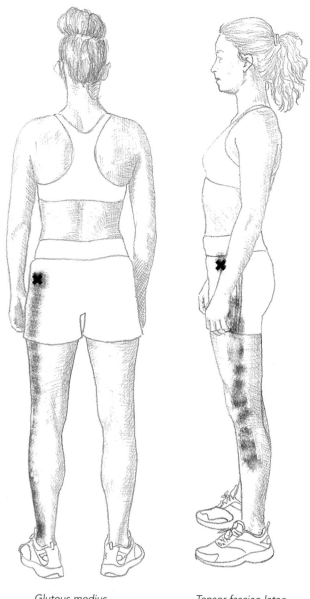

Gluteus medius   Tensor fasciae latae

The X marks the position of the trigger point, and the colored area indicates the possible spread of discomfort.

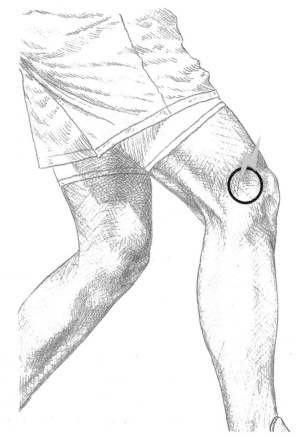

Runner's knee is a condition that responds very well to stretching.

General Remedies

If you're experiencing pain, avoid running, walking, or biking. Feel free to exercise, but stop as soon as you feel discomfort.

Specific Remedies

Stretch the following muscles several times a day, as well as before and after workouts.

When to Seek Professional Help

See a professional if the pain turns into chronic ache.

Muscles to Stretch

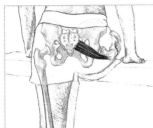

Piriformis, pages 72, 75

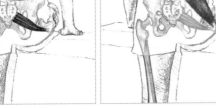

Gluteus medius and minimus, page 70

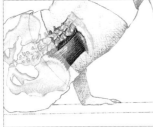

Quadratus lumborum, pages 78, 81

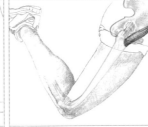

Tensor fasciae latae, page 92

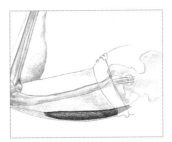

Rectus femoris, pages 86, 90

LOWER-BACK PAIN

Most people will have pain in the lower back at some point. In addition to personal suffering and a decline in quality of life, this ailment costs society an incredible amount of money in terms of missed work, sick days, and disability pay.

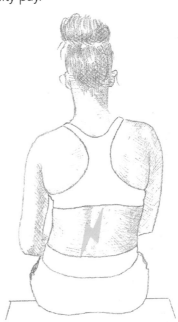

Sitting is one of the best ways to cause lower-back pain. Sitting while crossing your legs further increases the risk of hurting your back.

What Hurts?

- The discs in the spine
- Ligaments
- Immobilized joints in the spine and hip
- Joints in the spine and hip that are hypermobilized
- Tight muscles that spasm

Background

There are a multitude of reasons for lower-back pain. The main reason is that we sit too much, too long, and for too many years, compressing the discs in the spine and stretching out the ligaments. Sitting also tightens and shortens the hip flexors and the gluteal muscles and fatigues the deep muscles in the lower back.

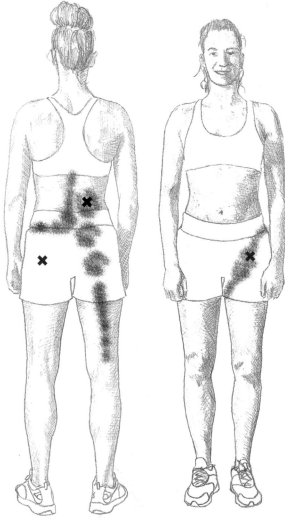

Iliopsoas—red ×
Quadratus lumborum—black ×
Piriformis—green ×

The X marks the position of the trigger point and the colored area indicates the possible spread of discomfort.

General Remedies

Avoid sitting, which lessens the activation of the muscles. Try to move rather often for short periods of time throughout the day. Sitting in front of the computer for hours and hours is devastating for the back.

Specific Remedies

Stretch the following muscles several times a day.

When to Seek Professional Help

See a professional if you have any of the following:

- Aching or pain so severe that you cannot sleep
- Pain that does not change throughout the day or with a shift in position
- Strong pain that radiates into the leg, lower leg, and foot
- Loss of strength in the leg
- Inability to stand on the toes or heels without sinking down
- Stabbing feeling in the back and leg when you sneeze or cough

Muscles to Stretch

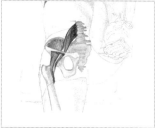
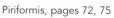

Piriformis, pages 72, 75

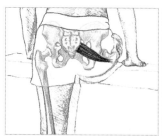

Psoas and iliacus, page 83

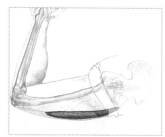

Rectus femoris, pages 86, 90

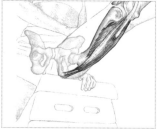

Hamstrings, page 95

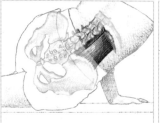

Quadratus lumborum, pages 78, 81

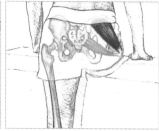

Gluteus medius and minimus, page 70

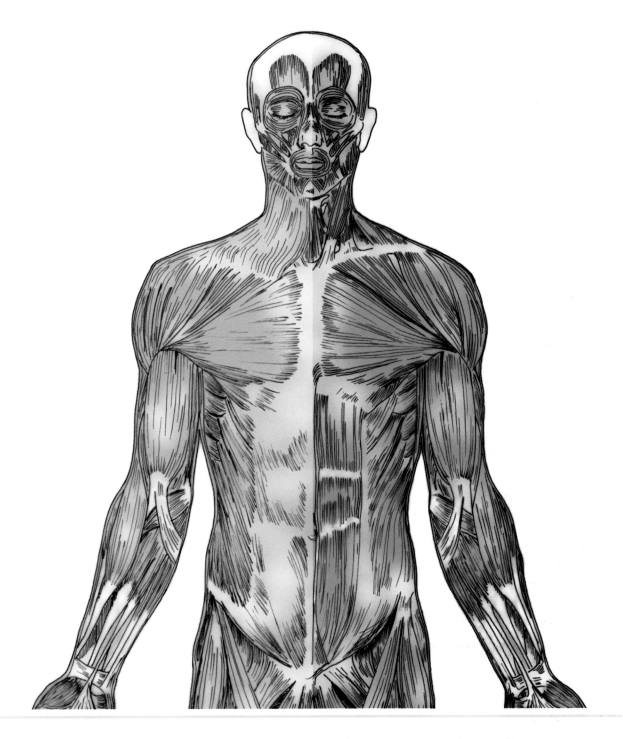

ASSESSING FLEXIBILITY
AND MUSCLE BALANCE

Lots of aches, pains, and injuries develop due to an imbalance of flexibility between the muscles on your left and right sides. The difference does not have to be great to cause real problems. When testing your flexibility, do not force yourself to stretch as far as you can. Instead, stop when you feel resistance, or stinging, in the muscle. This sensation should be the same on both sides. Remember to perform the exercises in the same way for each side.

Muscle being stretched	Shorter on left side	Shorter on right side	Equal
TEST FOR THE NECK AND SHOULDER			
Upper trapezius			
Levator scapulae			
Sternocleidomastoid			
Scalenes			
TEST FOR THE SHOULDER JOINT			
Supraspinatus			
Infraspinatus			
Teres major			
Latissimus dorsi			
TEST FOR THE UPPER BACK			
Middle trapezius			
Rhomboids			
Latissimus dorsi			
Pectoralis major			
TEST FOR THE LOWER BACK			
Psoas and iliacus			
Piriformis			
Gluteus medius and minimus			
Rectus femoris			
Hamstrings			

From K. Berg, 2011, *Prescriptive Stretching* (Champaign, IL: Human Kinetics).

STRETCH INDEX

REFERENCES

Amako, M., T. Oda, K. Masuoka, H. Yokoi, and P. Campisi. 2003. Effect of static stretching on prevention of injuries for military recruits. *Military Medicine* 168: 442-446.

Barcsay, Jenö. 1976. *Anatomy for artists.* [Anatomi för konstnärer.] Stockholm: Bonnier.

Bojsen-Möller, Finn. 2000. *The anatomy of the musculoskeletal system.* [Rörelseapparatens anatomi.] Stockholm: Liber.

Feland, J.B., J.W. Myrer, S.S. Schulthies, G.W. Fellingham, and G.W. Measom. 2001. The effect of duration of stretching of the hamstring muscle group for increasing range of motion in people aged 65 years or older. *Physical Therapy* 81: 1110-1117.

Fowles, J.R., D.G. Sale, and J.D. MacDougall. 2000. Reduced strength after passive stretch of the human plantar-flexors. *Journal of Applied Physiology* 89: 1179-1188.

Halbertsma, J.P., Al van Bolhuis, and L.N. Göeken. 1996. Sport stretching: Effect on passive muscle stiffness on short hamstrings. *Archives of Physical Medicine and Rehabilitation* 77: 688-692.

Harvey, L., R. Herbert, and J. Crosbie. 2002. Does stretching induce lasting increases in joint ROM? A systematic review. *Physiotherapy Research International* 7: 1-13.

Handel, M., T. Horstmann, H.H. Dickhuth, and R.W. Gulch. 1997. Effects of contract-relax stretching training on muscle performance in athletes. *European Journal of Applied Physiology and Occupational Physiology* 76: 400-408.

Karlsson, T., and M. Hallonlöf. 2003. *Stretching the hamstrings: The effect on quadriceps femoris regarding strength.* [Stretching av hamstrings: Effekt på quadriceps femoris beträffande styrka.] Stockholm: Karolinska Institute.

Lundeberg, Thomas, and Ralph Nisell. 1993. *Pain and inflammation: Physiology and pain in the moving parts.* [Smärta och inflammation: fysiologi och behandling vid smärta i rörelseorganen.] Stockholm: Syntex Nordica.

Peterson, Florence P., Elizabeth Kendall McCreary, and Patricia Geise Provance. 1993. *Muscles, testing and function: With posture and pain.* Baltimore: Williams & Wilkins.

Petrén, Ture. 1989. *Textbook of anatomy: Musculoskeletal system.* [Lärobok i anatomi: Rörelseapparaten.] Stockholm: Nordic Bookstore.

Pope, R.P., R.D. Herbert, J.D. Kirwan, and B.J. Graham. 2000. A randomized trial of preexercise stretching for prevention of lower limb injury. *Medicine and Science in Sports and Exercise* 32: 271-277.

Putz, R., and R. Pabst, eds. 2001. *Sobotta atlas of human anatomy: Head, neck, upper limb.* Munich: Elsevier, Urban & Fischer.

Putz, R., and R. Pabst, eds. 2001. *Sobotta atlas of human anatomy: Trunk, viscera, lower limb.* Munich: Elsevier, Urban & Fischer.

Richer, Paul. 1971. *Artistic anatomy.* trans. Robert Beverly Hale. New York: Watson-Guptill.

Rohen, Johannes W., Chihiro Yokochi, and Elke Lütjen-Drecoll. 1998. *Color atlas of anatomy: A photographic study of the human body.* Baltimore: Williams & Wilkins.

Szunyoghy, András. 1999. *Anatomical drawing school: Humans, animals, comparative anatomy.* [Anatomisk tecknarskola människa, djur, jämförande anatomi.] London: Könemann.

Travell, Janet G., David G. Simons, and Lois S. Simons. 1999. *Myofascial pain and dysfunction: The trigger point manual.* Baltimore: Williams & Wilkins.